SPECIAL PRAISE FOR

wild & well

"We lead interconnected lives. Dani expertly unpacks why we can't think about our health in isolation—and why the best solution isn't always more medication. If you're ready for a holistic, practical approach to your health, read on."

MICHAEL HYATT

New York Times *bestselling author*

"With a few Google searches, anyone can easily discover which foods are inflammatory or what doctors say about getting adequate rest. But I believe people resonate with a book for far more than its content. I believe people will resonate with this book because of its overarching and undeniable message of hope. If you have been feeling broken—physically, emotionally, mentally— Dani will let you know that you are not alone. You also don't have to stay that way!

Dani's six steps are part of the prescription that she gives every single one of her patients who are suffering from autoimmune disease, lifestyle diseases, and more that lead to strained relationships and exhaustion. You are not sinking, and you are stronger than you know, and I know you will be inspired to living your wildest and most well life thanks to Dani's wit, wisdom, and research."

JJ VIRGIN

Four-Time NYT bestselling author, Celebrity Nutrition & Fitness Expert

"Dani Williamson is a force of nature. And now she has taken that force and combined it with science, motivation and tools, cooked it all up in an easily digestible book that gives you answers, hope, and laughter.

I have known Dani for a number of years. I often teach MDs, NPs and pharmacists continuing medical education courses. We met there and it was instant sisters-of-the heart. Dani is one of the hardest working functional health care practitioners in the business. She has heart. Plus smarts. This book will give you heart + smart, too!

In this book you Dani gives it to you straight. And with this easy read, you get a large tool bag. Tools are the bomb! I have been in functional medicine for many decades and seen and heard many practitioners. You want someone that walks their talk and then helps you soar with yours. This book is that."

DR. DEVAKI LINDSEY BERKSON
Founder of drlindseyberkson.com (books, podcast and blog), Dr. Berkson's Best Health Radio, and female hormone line with Biotics (Receptor Detox and Hormone Daily Protector)

"Dani Williamson is the embodiment of *Wild and Well!* Her fiery red hair, open heart and compassion for the wellness and wellbeing of others shines in absolutely everything she says and does. She walks the walk and knows how to get you there too! If you want to look and feel amazing inside and out and regain the vibrant life you once had or always dreamed of having, read this transformational book and learn from my friend who's been down the road and back again and is stronger because of it."

DR. ANNA CABECA, OB/GYN
Bestselling author of The Hormone Fix and Keto-Green 16

"Remembering to take care of yourself is hard. And as simple as the self-care solutions may seem, how many of us actually feel inspired to practice them? What I love about Dani and her new book, *Wild and Well*, is how unbelievably doable and attainable she makes it all! Get ready to be inspired by Dani and her wellness leadership model to jump into action in order to reclaim your health and happiness!"

HAYLEY HUBBARD
Co-founder of Meaning Full Living & Mom of 3

"A workbook and a wakeup call, loaded with tips and tidbits, Dani takes on the vital role of challenging our ingrained belief systems and offering an opportunity to change course. Dani does a stellar job of pulling back the self-limiting curtain of our perception and illuminating a new thoughtful and hopeful path forward. Dani walks us down memory lane of how and why we have arrived at this moment of medical mayhem fraught with fragmentation, dysfunction and rampant failure. But she also inspires us with her wild and wellness-centric ways to both individually and collectively do what is innately possible, to rebel against a broken system and to create a new reality beyond only surviving, but thriving."

DR. NASHA WINTERS, ND, FABNO
Founder and CEO, drnasha.com

"Dani is a true warrior and a meaningful advocate for helping you navigate your best and most vibrant life. We all have missteps, and we have have struggles. We learn from each other! It is what you do in the face of those struggles that matter the most to me. If you want to heal and regain your health for good, FOR LIFE, I highly recommend this book. She is the real deal!"

TYLER HUBBARD
Florida Georgia Line

"Dani Williamson has captured and exquisitely articulated the power of self-care, self-love and empowerment to heal and regain the vibrant life you deserve and desire. Dani's incomparable spirit and dedicated compassion is apparent on every page throughout this must-read book. Filled with practical, realistic and insightful stories and strategies, you can't help being inspired to do all you can to embrace Dani's signature pillars of health. The message is clear, as she shares her hard-earned wisdom inspired by her personal journey. I know I'll be relying on the book as a resource for my personal healing as well as those I guide on their journeys to sustainable recovery."

MINDY GORMAN-PLUTZER FNLP, CEPC, CHC
Functional Nutrition and Eating Psychology Coaching

wild & well

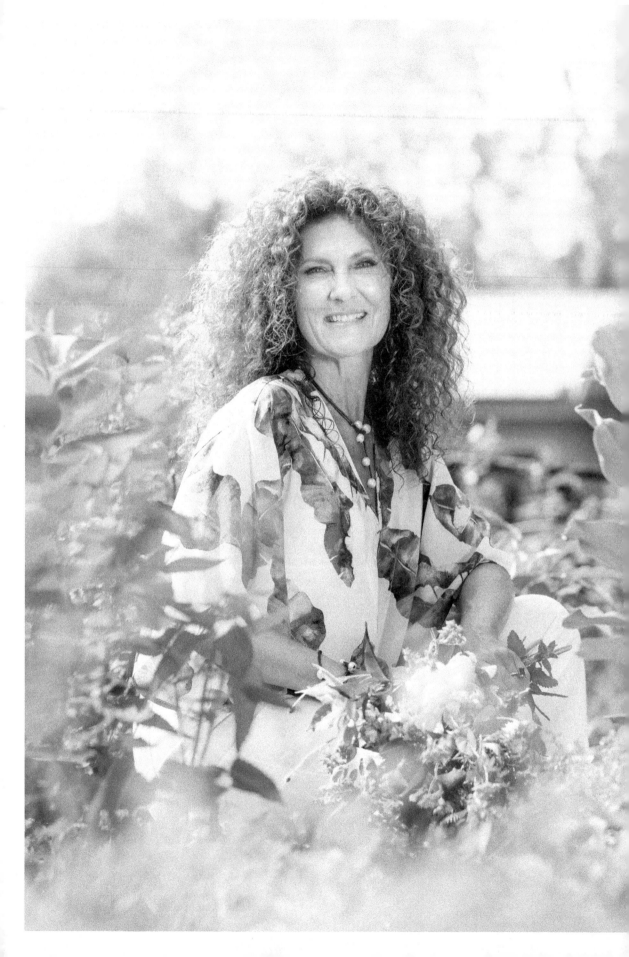

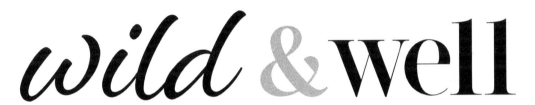

wild & well

Dani's Six Commonsense Steps to Radical Healing

DANI WILLIAMSON, MSN, FNP

WITH JENNIFER LILL BROWN

Foreword by Dr. Josh Axe

NEW YORK

LONDON • NASHVILLE • MELBOURNE • VANCOUVER

wild & well

Dani's Six Commonsense Steps to Radical Healing

THE HOLY BIBLE, NEW INTERNATIONAL VERSION®, NIV® Copyright © 1973, 1978, 1984, 2011 by Biblica, Inc.™ Used by permission. All rights reserved worldwide.

Published In New York, New York, by Morgan James Publishing. Morgan James is a trademark of Morgan James, LLC. www.MorganJamesPublishing.com

For more information contact:

Integrative Family Medicine
330 Mallory Station Rd, Unit B3
Franklin, TN 37067
info@daniwilliamson.com
Tel: 615.944.3530

DaniWilliamson.com
Instagram: @daniwilliamsonwellness
YouTube: Dani Williamson Wellness
Facebook: Join our private group
"Inside Out - Healing From Within"

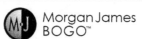

Morgan James
BOGO™

A **FREE** ebook edition is available for you
or a friend with the purchase of this print book.

CLEARLY SIGN YOUR NAME ABOVE

Instructions to claim your free ebook edition:
1. Visit MorganJamesBOGO.com
2. Sign your name CLEARLY in the space above
3. Complete the form and submit a photo
   of this entire page
4. You or your friend can download the ebook
   to your preferred device

ISBN 9781631955594 paperback
ISBN 9781631955617 ebook
ISBN 9781631955600 hardcover
Library of Congress Control Number:
2021935745

Cover & Interior Design by:
Marisa Jackson

Cover & Interior Photos by:
Daniel C. White Photography
www.DanielCWhite.com

Cover photo location:
Fernvale Herban Flower Farm
owned by Cindy Shapton
The Cracked Pot Gardener
@thecrackpotgardener

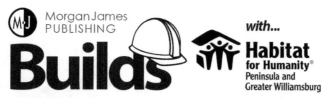

Morgan James is a proud partner of Habitat for Humanity Peninsula
and Greater Williamsburg. Partners in building since 2006.

Get involved today! Visit
MorganJamesPublishing.com/giving-back

This book is dedicated to

JACKSON AND ELLA

You are my heart and my soul. I'm honored to
be your mama. Stay Wild & Well, my loves.

table of
contents

acknowledgments

Seven years ago, my friend Michael Hyatt encouraged me to write a book—a book that would be a message of hope and healing to more than just one patient at a time. Seven years later, you are holding the final product of a true labor of love. I hope you love it as much as I do. I am a living example of how you can reverse the disease process. I want you to know that you are NOT broken, you were NEVER broken, and your body is designed to heal itself. You simply need a plan, and I have that for you.

This book would not be possible without so many people, too many to mention:

To my four best friends that I have had for decades, who are the true definition of community. Margo, Trish, Kim, and Billie—you are the roots that keep me standing and hold me accountable.

To my incredible office staff that is truly a "dream team."

To my community in Middle Tennessee that show up, show out, and share your life with me.

To Jen Lill Brown for putting my words so beautifully to paper and pressing on to get this book to print.

To Morgan James Publishing for taking a chance on an unknown author. I won't let you down.

To Mom, your life was never easy. Alzheimer's has taken its toll on you. I wish we could have known each other better. I will make the most of whatever time we have left to learn about each other.

To Dad and DeeDee, let's get the RV geared up for the Wild & Well Book Tour! Thanks for always being there for me.

Hang in there, ladies and gentlemen, because the best is yet to come! You got this.

Stay Wild & Well,

foreword

I have always believed that food is our greatest and most powerful medicine, just as Hippocrates once said. That is one of the reasons I was so intrigued when I first heard Dani Williamson's story. I know that food was her greatest *enemy* her entire life until the *one* day when someone she trusted spoke the words that changed her life forever: "Dani, what have you been eating? Don't you know that food determines your health?"

I first met Dani over ten years ago when she worked at Cool Springs Family Medicine, in Franklin, Tennessee, where I'd stop by to drop off copies of my first book, *The Real Food Diet*. I've since watched her take the leap of faith and start her own now-thriving practice, Integrative Family Medicine, in Franklin.

I have seen her passion and know she cares about not just *helping* people, but rather transforming them. That is precisely why, when I come across a complicated case (a person who other doctors keep reassuring, "Your labs are normal… you'll be just fine" but they *know* they are not fine), I send them to Dani.

She WAS that patient. She's been on the receiving end of one careless diagnosis after another, and it wasn't until she realized the power of food that her life was also transformed.

Dani is the real deal, and I trust her approach because she works on healing from the inside-out. She is my go-to source for healing from many auto-immune diseases, and I've even brought her into Ancient Nutrition to do a lunch and learn on Hashimoto's.

Dani is as bold as her hair, and her fearlessness is unrivaled. Listen to her wisdom, learn from her mistakes, benefit from her knowledge, and reclaim the vitality and joy that you deserve! I pray that *Wild and Well* and its straightforward steps to transformational healing will change the trajectory of your life and your family's lives.

—Dr. Josh Axe, DNM, DC, CNS
Author of *Ancient Remedies*

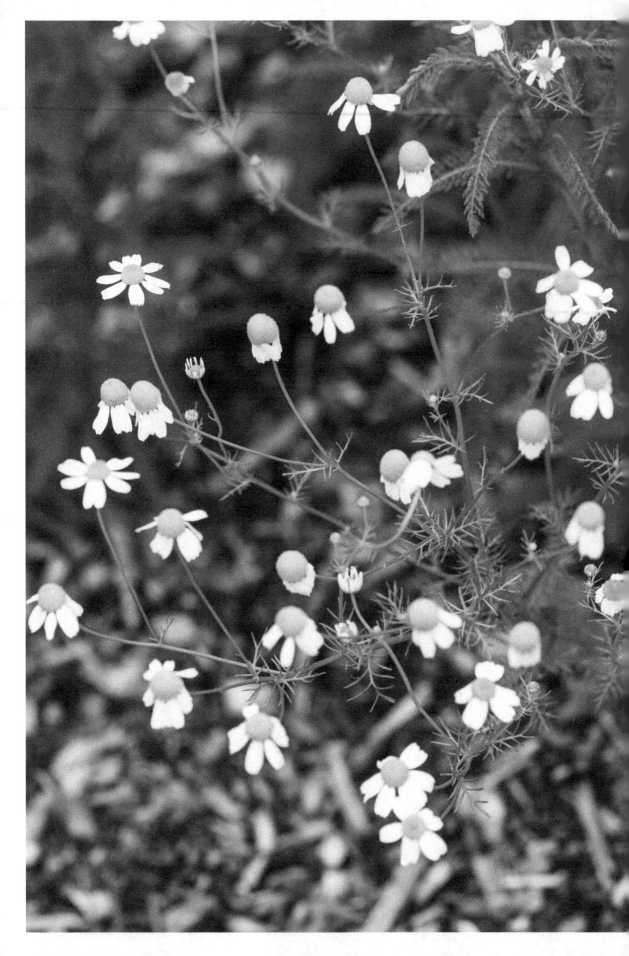

PART ONE

commonsense
evidence

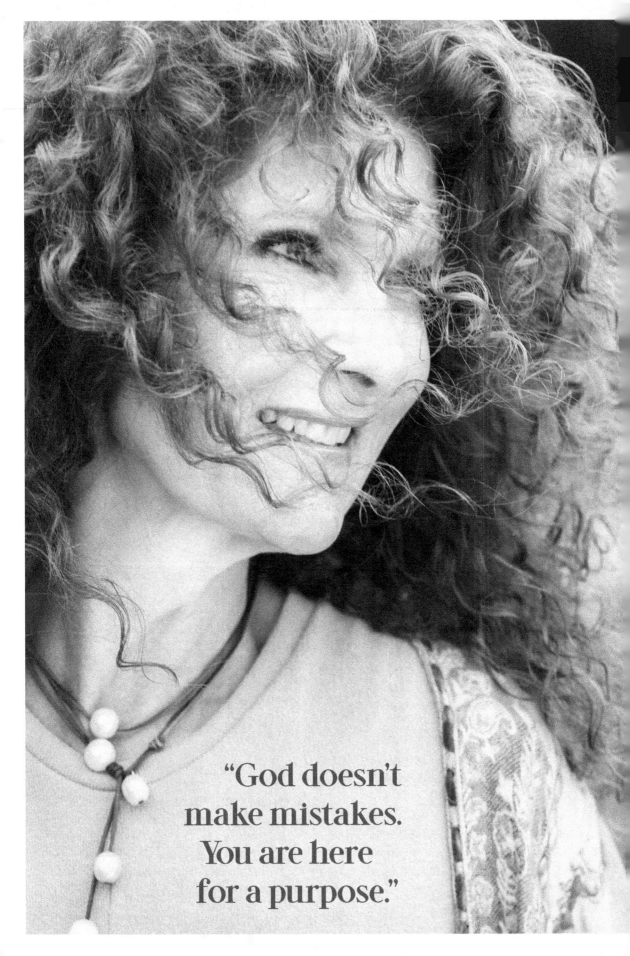

"God doesn't
make mistakes.
You are here
for a purpose."

you are not sinking

*"Be careful about reading health books.
You may die of a misprint."*

MARK TWAIN

In a time when we have access to more knowledge and resources than ever before, and we hold the power of information *literally* in the palm of our hands, a strange thing is happening:

We still believe most of what we hear.

Maybe we do this because it's easier for our brains to file things away quickly so we can get back to speeding through life. Who in the world has the time to dig more deeply? We barely have time to sleep!

If you have never stopped to question traditional medical professionals or universal truths until now, then welcome to the club! You are now a part of a tribe of human beings who no longer accept answers that don't add up. It took me most of my life to get to a place where "that's just the way it is" and "all of your labs are normal" don't cut it anymore.

As awake as you are, I can probably guess a few universal truths you might still believe. Let's see if any of these sounds familiar:

> My body is broken. I have an autoimmune disease, and I will have it for the rest of my life.
>
> I wish I had the energy of my younger years, but as we get older, we get tired. That's just the way it is. I need coffee to function, and I'm ashamed that I go back to sleep after the kids get on the bus.
>
> I struggle to fall asleep, and then I struggle to stay asleep. With the stresses of career, kids, and life, my brain stays on overdrive. That's just the way it is.
>
> When I was younger, I could eat whatever I wanted. Now, it doesn't matter what I do. That scale will not budge! My metabolism isn't what it used to be.
>
> Hormones wreak havoc on my body and mood every month. I'm so unpredictable! Things just haven't been the same since my pregnancies, and they never will be.
>
> Of course, I'm tired. I have three kids!
>
> Of course, I'm gaining weight. I'm not 21 anymore.
>
> Of course, I don't want to have sex anymore. That happens to everyone.
>
> Of course, I'm stressed out. Who isn't?

If you can relate to a few of these or all of them, you are not alone. Sadly, these supposed truths are lies that have kept us stuck not in a *healthcare* system, but in a *sick-care* system that frankly doesn't profit from happy, healthy patients.

I can tell from the conversations I have with patients, day-in and day-out, that most of us (myself included) feel like we are dog paddling, just trying to keep our heads above water. We juggle all the things—children, spouse, job, family, work, and social commitments. At some point, we start going through the motions. That's when we lose sight of the precious life that we've worked so hard to build.

I was so stressed when my children were small that I don't even remember most of their childhood. I was too consumed with perfection and trying to "do it all" to stop and soak up the joy.

I have since learned that you can't do it all and do it well. Something has to give, and most of the time, your marriage, your relationship with your children, and your health will yield first. Once you sprinkle in chronic illness, autoimmune disease, anxiety, depression, migraine headaches, hormone imbalances, heartburn, constipation, joint pain, insomnia, and weight gain, paddling becomes even more labored. That's when you feel like you're starting to drown, but let me tell you:

You are *not* sinking.

I know it may feel like you are already halfway under, but you are not. Another birthday does not automatically equal a new health condition, another ache, another pain, or another few pounds on the scale. Modern medicine is the thing that's broken, not your divinely designed body.

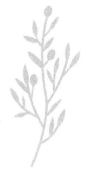

Modern medicine is the thing that's broken, not your divinely designed body.

You were designed to walk on water, just like Peter did as he walked toward Jesus on the Sea of Galilee. When I opened my practice, Integrative Family Medicine, in 2014, I stepped out of the boat on faith. I fixed my eyes on Jesus and kept walking. I believe you also have the courage to step out and walk toward Him.

Your past does not predict your future. Your past failures in eating well, exercising, trying to get enough sleep, and decreasing stress do not have to dictate your tomorrow. But you must first believe in yourself and keep your focus and your hope.

Hope is *not* a strategy—but it is a foundation for the right approach. I have written this book as a strategy for moving forward and living the life that God designed you to live. You deserve the truth, and you need the steps you can take *now* to break the chains of established wisdom and find freedom in total health!

I know what kind of person you are. You've done your research. You've tried over-the-counter (OTC) pills and prescription meds. You've seen specialists (the gastroenterologist, neurologist, rheumatologist, gynecologist, endocrinologist, and psychiatrist), and you asked them a straightforward question:

"Isn't there something I can do?"

The conventional answer you received is, "No. All of your labs are normal. But you should try to eat better and exercise more." Or maybe you heard, "You are probably just depressed. Let's try this anti-depressant and see how you feel."

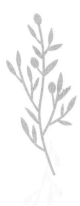

In most doctors' offices, you'll continue to receive stopgap medications that eventually make things worse.

However, the real answer is, **"Yes! There is so much you can do!"**

Your problems are not in your head.

There are decades of research to support the fact that not all solutions are found inside a prescription bottle. What the research *does* tell us is that autoimmune conditions often begin with inflammation and gut dysfunction.[1] Research tells us that gluten is inflammatory and a significant factor in the autoimmune thyroid crisis in this country.[2] Research tells us that type 2 diabetes can be reversed through dietary changes.[3] Research tells us that prolonged use of pharmaceuticals such as benzodiazepines causes a significantly higher risk of cognitive decline.[4]

I could go on and on—and we will continue to discuss what the research says about your health and how much control you have throughout this book. But you won't hear these kinds of facts inside the walls of modern exam rooms.

In most doctors' offices, you'll continue to receive stopgap medications that eventually make things worse.

"You have migraines? Must be an Imitrex deficiency. I'll write a prescription for you."

"Joint paint? Must be an NSAID deficiency. Take your Ibuprofen."

"Feeling anxious? Must be a Xanax deficiency. Here you go."

"Can't sleep? Must be an Ambien deficiency. This ought to do it."

But why does this happen? Believe it or not, we weren't taught to treat root causes in nurse practitioner school. Instead, we were taught to suppress symptoms and to give the *illusion* of healing, not actual healing. In defense of my gifted professors, I am not sure they realized that what they were teaching us is not healing medicine. They taught what they had been taught because that's how traditional allopathic school operates.

The thing is, "because we've always done it this way" is not a sufficient answer for me anymore. True healing is found in discovering and treating root causes. Treating symptoms is a Band-Aid approach.

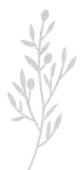

Numb the pain all you want, but the root will still be there when the meds wear off.

A headache is many times a symptom of the root cause, not the mechanism to treat or heal. Joint pain is a symptom of what's actually going on in your body. **Numb the pain all you want, but the root will still be there when the meds wear off.** From atherosclerosis and metabolic disorders to lung cancer and more, the research shows that underlying causes for symptoms could extend as far back as in utero.[5,6,7]

When I realized that my story is similar to many of the patients that I see daily, I knew I needed to write a book to help people, not just in my clinic, but worldwide. There is a root cause for nearly every condition—and my story is proof of this fact.

There's a Pill for That

I grew up in a small Western Kentucky town called Gilbertsville, just outside of Paducah, where chemical plants along the Tennessee River spew out toxins around the clock. My dad worked in one of those plants for many years before buying a small hamburger restaurant in town. The irony of my family owning a greasy spoon for 28 years that serves inflammatory foods like hamburgers, French fries, and ice cream does not escape me. Although he did get his hamburger meat fresh every day from the local butcher, I feel certain it wasn't organic, grass-fed, or hormone-free.

In my practice, one of the first things we dig into is family history—emotional abuse, verbal abuse, divorce, and other childhood traumas. Your past is a significant part of your story. It plays an influential role in how you feel about yourself and virtually every choice you make. Your body keeps score of your past traumas and experiences, whether you want it to or not.

I had a rather traumatic, highly stressful adolescence. My parents got divorced when I was in second grade, and my mom married a man who turned out to be a child molester. Her next husband was verbally and emotionally abusive and became physically abusive during my senior year of high school.

I started working at 13 to escape my house for a few more hours a day. I worked two, sometimes three jobs during high school, and I pushed myself so hard that I caught mono during my junior year. I was miserably homebound as I recovered.

I struggled with gut issues for as long as I can remember. I felt stressed beyond belief, and it affected the way I interacted with the world around me. I remember once at a local pharmacy when I was 15, the man behind the counter looked down at me and said, "Smile! It can't be that bad."

But it really was that bad.

My mom was on her third marriage at the time and was more miserable than I was. How could that *not* affect a child? I should have been laughing and having the time of my life, but the mask I wore to keep the truth about my home life a secret weighed me down.

I left for college at Western Kentucky University and joined a sorority. I felt free for the first time, but my body would soon have other plans. My gut was a mess, and, at age 20, I had my first colonoscopy. The diagnosis was a spastic colon, which is an old term for what we now call irritable bowel syndrome, or IBS.

I was prescribed Librax, a medication that's supposed to help decrease gastrointestinal motility and soothe extreme digestive upset. Unfortunately, it is a benzodiazepine (benzo for short), which is a class of drugs originally designed to treat anxiety disorders. Benzos are known for their calming effect, so much so that they are frequently used to help sedate nervous patients before surgery.

I went to work at Western's financial aid department the following day, but I was so sluggish that I couldn't function. I took Librax for two days and then abruptly threw the bottle away. I never wanted to feel like that again.

At that point, I had no idea what benzodiazepines were and how addictive they are. Recent research has shown that benzos are not even the best medications for a spastic colon.[8] It's a class of medications that I refuse to prescribe to my patients for any reason whatsoever.

My symptoms persisted, thanks to constant stress and an inflammatory diet. The bloating, gas, chronic diarrhea, and stomach pain were making life unbearable. I went to three different gastroenterologists who essentially treated me like a lab rat. One medicine wouldn't work, so they'd pull me off that and prescribe another one in its place.

Did anyone ever ask about my home life or stress levels? Of course not. Did my doctors ever ask me what I was eating? Not once. If they had, I could have just shown them a photo of my sorority sisters and I holding giant bags of onion rings, French fries, and corn dogs that my dad had sent with me to college.

No one ever asked me anything other than, "What symptoms are you experiencing right now?"

This is because the medical system operates with flawed methods by treating *dysfunction* rather than *pathology*.

The medical system operates with flawed methods by treating *dysfunction* rather than *pathology*.

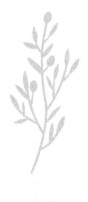

Thanks to my "mystery symptoms" that would have been obvious to any respectable functional medicine doctor, I underwent more invasive testing. After my original colonoscopy, I had an endoscopy (a nonsurgical procedure to examine the GI tract), a barium enema (an x-ray of the large intestine), and a barium swallow (an x-ray to explore the upper GI tract). I also ended up having three more colonoscopies that never led to any real answers—only more ineffective treatments.

They put me on all the proton pump inhibitors, including Nexium, Prilosec, and Protonix, which are designed to treat heartburn and acid reflux, or GERD. No one ever told me that one of the side effects of drugs like Protonix is diarrhea![9] Proton pump inhibitors are shown to lower stomach acid levels so much that it allows a harmful bacterium called C. difficile (typically kept in check by stomach acid) to proliferate and cause chronic diarrhea.[10]

In short, not only were the medications ineffective, but, in many cases, they were making things worse. When that happened, I was told to take Mylanta and TUMS as often as needed.

My symptoms increased exponentially during my pregnancies, especially the heartburn. I have a priceless photo of me lying on the couch on Thanksgiving of 1995 with a bottle of Mylanta balanced on my giant pregnant belly. I vividly remember asking my obstetrician if it was possible to take too much Mylanta.

One day, I started itching uncontrollably and didn't stop. My lower arms and upper legs were red, prickly, irritated, and scaly from my late twenties into my thirties. I would lie in bed, scratching my arms and legs so forcefully that I would find blood on the sheets in the morning. Sometimes I'd wake up in the middle of the night and wrap ice packs around my arms and cold dishcloths around my legs in an attempt to stop the itching enough to get some rest.

I used Benadryl for a long time. Unfortunately, no one ever told me that long-term use of anticholinergic drugs like Benadryl causes permanent neurological effects such as memory loss and dementia.[11,12,13] As a person with dementia and mental health issues in her family, I would have liked to know that.

I saw two dermatologists who used steroids as a temporary fix to at least make me functional. The steroids did their job and decreased my inflammation. Using them was the only thing that enabled me to work and operate as a business owner and parent.

Unfortunately, the dermatologists never connected my gut health to my skin health. As the largest organ, the skin is the window to internal health.[14] I tell patients every day that their eczema, dermatitis, psoriasis, chronic itching (urticaria), or acne most likely has a direct correlation to gut dysfunction.[15,16] Heal the gut and, more often than not, the skin will also heal.[17] We can attribute this to emerging evidence that shows the presence of a line of communication in the body, referred to as the gut-skin axis.[18,19]

Two highly respected dermatologists entirely missed this straightforward concept. Every day when I look at those scars on my arms and upper legs, I think about all those years of misery. It saddens me that no one ever even suspected my skin issues could be linked to an unhealthy microbiome.

As if a spastic colon and chronic itching weren't enough, I started to feel increasingly agonizing joint pain, particularly in my hands and wrists. My short little fingers looked like sausages when I woke up in the mornings, and my thumb pads would get so swollen and painful that I could hardly shake hands.

I owned a maternity store called Mum's the Word, and I was raising two small children in an unhealthy marriage. I was already exhausted from the pace of life and lack of sleep. On top of that, I had to deal with constant bloating, chronic diarrhea, uncontrollable itching, and hands that didn't want to work anymore.

I told my OB-GYN about my joint symptoms, and she decided to run some tests. I'll never forget the day she called and asked if she could come by the house to discuss the results. She sat me down and said in disbelief, "These labs say you have lupus, Dani."

I shrugged. "Well, I told you I didn't feel good."

My doctor had her doubts and wanted to re-draw my blood. She couldn't accept that the results were correct because my antibodies were so elevated. The only person I knew with lupus was my ex-husband's cousin, who was my hairdresser. I had watched her struggle with the disease for years, so I hoped there was a mistake.

There was no mistake. My antibodies were even higher the second time. I was immediately referred to Vanderbilt to see "the best rheumatologist in the region." Here is what she proceeded to tell me within five minutes of my first appointment:

> "There's no cure for lupus, Danielle. People die from this disease every year. Here are your pain meds and your anti-inflammatory drugs. These could damage your kidneys, though, so we'll need to check your kidneys and liver every six months."

I was horrified. The rheumatologist initially prescribed Vioxx for the pain, but I only took it for a few days. Even though I knew nothing about functional medicine or holistic health, I instinctively sensed that it was not good for me. I stopped the Vioxx on my own just like I did with the Librax years before. It's a good thing, too, since Vioxx was taken off the market worldwide shortly after that due to its link to increased risk of heart disease, heart attack, and stroke.[20,21] I could have easily been just another forgotten wrongful death lawsuit against a pharmaceutical giant.

Endings and Beginnings

I saw doctor after doctor for two long, excruciating decades. During this time, I functioned adequately in the outside world, and I also *looked* great. I owned my maternity store, taught yoga, raised kids, and even became a doula. I was doing all of the things I needed to do. I felt awful, but I gutted through it because I had to.

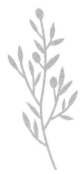

> I was paddling so frantically but continued to sink. Still, I knew I had to keep trying.

One day, I decided I couldn't take it anymore. For the first time, I completely understood how people could choose to end their own lives. My then-husband Greg had just left for work, and it was time for me to get up, feed the kids, and open my store.

I laid there unable to move, and I wondered if it might be time to end my suffering. I wanted to leave the world—but then I looked down at the foot of my bed and saw my two children standing there, and I knew I wasn't going anywhere.

I was paddling so frantically but continued to sink. Still, I knew I had to keep trying.

I found a psychologist in Nashville and drove two hours to visit her every week for months. She suggested to have a doctor write me a prescription for an anti-depressant, and I wasted no time in doing so. Over the next few years, I tried them all, from Lexapro and Effexor to Prozac and Paxil.

When these drugs deadened my mood and sex drive, that was the final nail in the coffin of my marriage that had been on life support for several years. We called it quits in 2003 after I admitted to a long, secret extramarital affair.

The marriage would never have lasted with or without my infidelity, but it didn't help matters. I humiliated my husband and created such a scandal in our small community. Hindsight being what it is, I know I should have left the marriage years before that happened—but all I can do is make better choices going forward.

I've asked God for forgiveness, and I've slowly learned to forgive myself. I also hope my ex-husband will forgive me someday.

As I mentioned, during my time as a business owner, I moonlighted as a yoga instructor, childbirth educator, and doula. In fact, I was the first certified doula in Western Kentucky, assisting in over 40 births. After close friends encouraged me to pursue nursing since I greatly enjoyed my doula work, I decided to start nursing school prerequisites with my friend Trish. I remember this like it was yesterday—Trish and I laugh often about the summer day we were lying on my bed talking about our futures (we were both recently divorced with three little kids between us). She and I looked at each other and said almost in tandem, "Let's go to nursing school together." Now, over 15 years later, we are both working in a field we love.

Though I had a lot going on at that point, my store had been struggling since September 11, 2001. Business as whole took a blow on that tragic day, and, sadly, my store never recovered. So, in 2004, I finally closed Mum's the Word Maternity Store, and I began teaching more yoga to pay the bills while I took classes.

It was a financially turbulent season, and eventually, I was forced to seek government aid. I remember the most *humiliating* day of my life like it was yesterday. My friend Margo and I walked into the food stamp office in Paducah. I was there to apply for State aid to feed my children, and Margo was there for moral support.

The woman sitting across the desk looked at me and said, "Aren't you Dani from Mum's the Word Maternity Store?"

Tears started streaming down my face, and I cried hysterically for several minutes, there in the office, with all eyes on me. Margo cried right along with me.

The five years I spent on food stamps was the hardest period of my life. But it helped to set the foundation for the time to come. That difficult season made me stronger and more determined to find a better way.

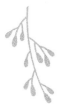

God had a plan during all those years of struggle.

I'll never forget one of the *proudest* moments of my life in January of 2006. I went to the mailbox to find two letters waiting for me. I opened the first letter that read, "Congratulations! You've been accepted into Vanderbilt University School of Nursing."

The second letter was from the Kentucky. It read, "Congratulations! You qualify for $56 more dollars a month in food stamps for you and your children."

I have both letters framed in my office as a reminder to my patients and me that no matter how close you feel you are to drowning, there is always a life preserver within reach.

God had a plan during all those years of struggle.

I had no idea what the future would hold, and, frankly, I'm glad I didn't. If I had known what I had yet to endure, I'm not sure I would have signed on for the wild ride.

I wasn't out of the woods yet. I was still dealing with chronic gut issues, a painful skin condition, depression, and autoimmune disease. Still, for the first time in a long time, I felt hope.

So, I had faith, reached out my hand, and stepped out of the boat. In May of 2006, I packed up a 26-foot U-Haul and drove it to Nashville, Tennessee, along with two small children, an aging dog, a cat, and two hermit crabs—and we started our lives over from scratch.

It was time to make some serious changes. I was done, but not with life. I was done accepting answers that didn't make sense, and I was done with conventional wisdom. I wanted to learn the truth.

The Question That Changed Everything

At Vanderbilt, we learned a lot of truths about the human body, but we also learned that health is found at the pharmacy. I knew it was the wrong answer. I knew it in my gut, which is ironic since that's where all of my problems started.

I accepted my first position before I'd even passed my boards. At the time, my son Jackson was living with my ex-husband, and I couldn't stand not seeing him regularly. So, Ella and I moved back to Western Kentucky, and I started working as a nurse practitioner in the ER of a local hospital.

I loved it! It was exhilarating for me to help with urgent care cases, and I was learning the job, having only 20 minutes of orientation on my first day. I loved the energy of the ER, and how fast paced the environment was.

Still, life has a way of showing you your correct path in ways you least expect. My sexist (this trait was well known throughout the hospital) boss called me into a room one day shortly after I started to give me some surprising and hard-to-believe news. "Dani," he said, "You're just not learning as fast as we want you to learn."

I was shocked. "But I love this job," I replied.

He shot back without missing a beat, "Dani, nobody loves this job. They only do it for the money. You can either work for another month or leave today and be paid for the month."

I handed him the chart that was in my hand for a toothache and walked out the door. I had just been fired—with almost $200,000 in student loans and living in a town I swore I'd never live in again.

It was January of 2010 (two months after being hired), and a magnitude 7 earthquake had just demolished Haiti. Something in my spirit said, "Go," and so I went. I spent 21 days in Haiti, living in a tent and helping the victims. I saw horrific things I'll never forget. I put my brief time in the Kentucky ER to good use by moving quickly and helping as many people as I could. I suppose part of it was my way of showing my former boss what a mistake he had made in firing me. I was reliable under pressure, and I knew my stuff.

Going to Haiti was life-changing for me and brought some much-needed clarity. I knew I wanted to help people in a real way and not just become a drug dispensary. After I returned home, I moved back to Nashville with my daughter Ella (Jackson came a few months later) to find a way to make that a reality.

In May of 2010, nearly a quarter of a century after my troubles began, a medical doctor finally asked me the right question that prompted my Eureka moment. I was working in a functional medicine office, and the owner of the clinic, Dr. Dan Kalb, quickly became the most exceptional teacher and mentor I have ever had.

One morning, I was filling him in on my extensive medical history. I laundry-listed all the drugs, all the diagnoses, all the pain, and all the years of frustration I had experienced as a patient in the traditional medical world.

Dr. Kalb was silent for a moment, and then he leaned in, looked me square in the eyes, and said:

"Dani, what are you eating?

Do you know your diet controls your symptoms?"

What? How had I not heard this before?

He asked me if I ever took digestive enzymes and probiotics, and if I knew my food sensitivities. "Food sensitivities? What does food have to do with IBS, skin issues, and autoimmune disease?"

As it turns out, food has *everything* to do with those conditions.

That day, Dr. Dan Kalb became my greatest mentor and the man who changed the entire trajectory of my life, my children's lives, and the lives of my patients. He began to teach me about holistic health, functional medicine, and the power of food. Even though I no longer work at Dr. Kalb's practice, he is still one of my biggest cheerleaders and mentors.

I had spent three years and $200,000 to receive a degree from one of the most highly respected nurse practitioner programs on the planet. Yet, not one time did they ever tell our class of over 300 students that our bodies are designed to heal themselves.

That our patients aren't born sick.

That food can be medicine.

Hippocrates, the father of medicine, once stated, "All disease begins in the gut." He also said, "Let food be your medicine and medicine be your food."

Somewhere along the way, our medical system lost sight of this ancient wisdom. We are in the business of sick care, not health care. During my brief stint in the ER, I learned that the goal was to "treat 'em and street 'em" as quickly as possible. Don't dig. Don't try to determine the root cause. Just catch and release.

I'll never be able to prove it, but I feel confident that if just *one* of my doctors had asked me about my diet, I never would have developed lupus. Instead, years of chronic, slow-burning inflammation turned IBS and itching into an autoimmune disease.

I wasn't born sick or fatigued. I wasn't born with chronic IBS or itching skin. I wasn't born with joint pain or lupus. Those conditions were the result of years of continual stress, poor diet, and nonexistent self-care.

> **God doesn't make garbage, and he doesn't make mistakes. You are here for a purpose.**

However, I'm also living, walking proof that what you turn on, you can turn back off again. Most of the lifestyle diseases we face in this country today—including many autoimmune conditions, hormone-related dysfunctions, heart disease, and obesity—are partially or even fully reversible.[22,23,24]

Remember, you are not sinking.

God's on your team, but that doesn't mean you get to lie back and float. You have to work, and you have to be willing to make significant changes. You can't change a few things and expect total health. You need to do a 180-degree turn and walk in an all-new direction. You also have to believe that you are worthy of being healthy and whole.

God doesn't make garbage, and he doesn't make mistakes. You are here for a purpose.

For my female readers: You play an integral role in your household by setting the tone. You choose what kind of nutrition your family consumes, what they allow into their minds, and what they value most, as well their overall outlook on health. It's a huge responsibility and one that I hope you do not take lightly. It also helps explain the fact that when you are overwhelmed and sick, it creates chaos and disruption in the home. I remember the days of chaos well, and I wish I could have a do-over—but that's not how life works.

Give yourself a break, and, for goodness sake, give yourself some grace! You provide plenty to others. Don't you deserve some, too? You are enough, and your body has the power to heal. Together with God, you and I are going to help you get your life back.

For my male readers: You are the rock and the foundation upon which your wife builds a happy, healthy home for your family. You've got to be your strongest, healthiest self on the inside before you can be what you need to be for anyone else!

Environment factors are the most significant detriments to your health—not genetics. Just because your family has a history of heart disease, diabetes, autoimmune disease, depression, anxiety, or obesity doesn't mean those conditions are inevitabilities for you. You may have certain genetic predispositions, but you don't have to turn on those genetics![25] We know this thanks to a field of study called epigenetics that we will discuss later in the book. The research tells us that gene transcription can be either *activated* or *inhibited* by environmental exposures, including food choices, sleep patterns, stress levels, and so much more.[26,27,28]

You are currently in one season of life out of many you will experience. Maybe you are getting ready for college or a new career. Perhaps you are a young mom struggling to keep your head above water with crying kids, lack of sleep, a neglected husband, and a dirty house. Maybe you are going through perimenopause or menopause, and it feels like you're going crazy. You might be caring for your aging parents as well as your family. You may be in a season of singleness and resent having to cook for one.

Regardless of where you are, stop and put your oxygen mask on FIRST because by saving yourself, you will be able to save others. When mom or dad feels better, the whole family feels better. If you don't have a family, then you are ahead of the game. Get yourself healthy before you have a spouse, children, or aging parents to balance.

Here's the Game Plan

This book is divided into two parts: commonsense evidence and common-sense action. In Part One, we will discuss topics like ACE (adverse childhood experience) testing and what I call *lifestyle diseases*. You will discover powerful, clear, and succinct information on what is causing you to feel the way you do. In Part Two, I'll spell out exactly what you can do about it! If you are ready to put on your gloves and fight, then consider Part Two as your coach that will get you ring-ready.

> A "normal" body is one that works the way God designed it to work.

My ultimate goal is to provide you with a commonsense guide to total restoration.

No matter what season you are in right now, I want to you be able to use the tools in this book to fight for the life God meant for you to have. I wrote it to give you hope and a strategy, but it's up to you to take it and run with it!

If you are suffering from autoimmune disease, thyroid issues, hormonal imbalance, weight gain, fatigue, bowel issues, low sex drive, insomnia, or stress, I've got you. It's not "normal" to put on weight and struggle to get it off. It's not "normal" for your body to have an autoimmune reaction. It's not "normal" to stop wanting to have sex with your spouse. It's not "normal" to have to take a pill to sleep.

A "normal" body is one that works the way God designed it to work.

I believe that the six steps on the path to health and healing are to eat well, sleep well, move well, poop well, de-stress well, and commune well. While I am passionate about these truths, I am even more excited about returning *your* passion for life to you. I hope to do that by helping you experience breakthroughs in your health that give your body and your health back.

It's your life, and you deserve to feel great! None of us know the moment we will take our final breath. Whether my last heartbeat comes today or 50 years from now, I want to be living my best life—inside and outside—at that moment.

When you are in pain, you are not suffering from a Tylenol deficiency. I will dispel the myths propagated by Band-Aid-style medicine and get to the root of your issues. Then, I will give you a precise plan for what to do and what not to do. I know what NOT to do because I've done it for most of my life.

People see health influencers and think we've got it all figured out. But I'm a work in progress, just like you! I'm not a magician or a world-renowned doctor. I'm just a country girl from Gilbertsville, Kentucky who had an epiphany one day. Someone finally looked me in the eyes and asked me the right questions, and now I get to share some research-based truths that will transform your life, if you are ready to have a little faith and step out of the boat.

wild & well Rx

Dani Williamson, MSN, FNP

R̶x

Patient Name: ....

Age: .... Date: ....

1. Believe that you are not broken, and you have never been broken.

2. Give your body what is needs to heal, because your body is designed to heal itself.

3. Know that you are worthy to begin this journey toward feeling Wild & Well.

4. Give yourself the grace that Jesus gives you and trust the journey.

5. Don't overdo it. Small, daily steps are the best way to approach healing for most.

6. Start with just one new action. If you are overwhelmed at the thought of even beginning, start with one thing.

7. Don't throw the baby out with the bathwater if you backslide! Get up and get back on the horse.

8. Keep it simple. Healing the body from the inside out is common sense and not complicated. Don't complicate the journey.

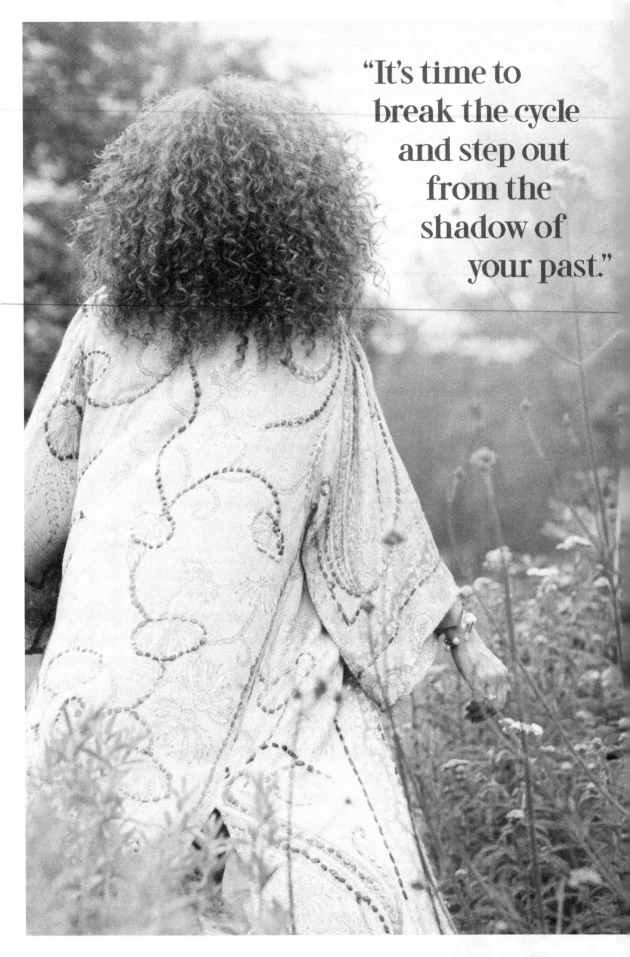

"It's time to break the cycle and step out from the shadow of your past."

you are not
your past

*"If you cannot get rid of the family skeleton,
you may as well make it dance."*
GEORGE BERNARD SHAW

Nothing messes you up quite like your childhood.

You just reacted to that statement somewhere in between "Amen to that!" and "No way, my childhood was amazing!"

Children are like lumps of clay that their parents have the responsibility to mold into something that functions well as an adult human being in the world. Some take this responsibility more seriously than others—either by instinct, by accident, or by choice.

Your parents raised you according to norms and principles upon which they were raised. They were products of their upbringing, and you are a product of yours. This type of reasoning provokes the "nature versus nurture" argument. How much about your lifestyle, choices, mindset, and health can you attribute to genes (nature), and how much can you attribute to environment (nurture)?

Just a few decades ago, the relationship between the brain and behavioral development was considered pretty cut and dry. Scientists believed that as the brain matures, it instinctively promotes healthy growth. Thanks to advances in neurobiological methods, however, we now know that it is the combination of genetic factors *and* the environment and experiences of each individual that guide brain development.[29]

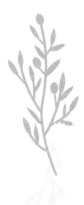

Common sense tells us that both nature and nurture matter when it comes to our health and future outcomes.

Common sense tells us that both nature and nurture matter when it comes to our health and future outcomes as well.

For example, recent research supports the fact that environmental factors (nurture) are more critical to gut microbiome ecology than host genetics (nature). In fact, unfavorable environmental factors are linked to a horde of adverse health responses, including the negative metabolic outcomes related to diabetes and obesity.[30]

Am I saying that genetics doesn't play a role in your health?

Of course not. What I *am* saying is that when it comes to your overall life direction and outcomes, genetics plays a secondary role to the environment in which you spent your youth.

In other words, I am talking about whether or not you had adverse childhood experiences.

Adverse Childhood Experiences

In 1995, the CDC partnered with healthcare titan Kaiser Permanente to conduct the Adverse Childhood Experiences (ACE) Study. The goal was to investigate childhood abuse, neglect, and other household challenges and their potential link to various problems in adult life.

Adverse childhood experiences or ACEs are stressful and traumatic events that occur in children's lives between the ages of 0 and 17. Examples include witnessing or experiencing violence or being abused mentally, physically, or sexually. ACEs also include environmental aspects that can damage a child's sense of stability and safety. These include substance abuse and mental health issues in the home, parental divorce, and incarceration of a family member.[31]

The ACE Study took more than two years to complete. It examined over 17,000 adult test subjects who received physical exams and took surveys regarding their childhood experiences and current health status and behaviors.

After the exhaustive study was complete, they concluded that 64 percent of the adult population had at least one ACE, and 12.5 percent of those people had four or more ACEs.[32] Some believe that the figures may be even higher since the study's participants were mostly white, college-educated, middle- and upper-middle-class Californians with excellent health care and good jobs.

> **Multiple, chronic, or persistent stress can impact a child's developing brain and has been linked to a variety of high-risk behaviors, chronic diseases, and unfavorable health outcomes in adulthood.**

The research also determined that ACEs are linked to chronic stress responses, much like the ones I experienced growing up that led to my IBS diagnosis at age 20. Multiple, chronic, or persistent stress can impact a child's developing brain and has been linked to a variety of high-risk behaviors, chronic diseases, and unfavorable health outcomes in adulthood.[33]

A growing number of medical doctors and counseling offices offer tests that can provide you with your "ACE score," which will typically be a number from 0 to 10. Additionally, there are numerous options to take the test online. The ten-question test requires only yes/no answers. So, are you ready to find out your ACE score? Here we go. Now turn the page and take the quick ACES quiz to find out your score.

Before your 18th birthday: Y/N

Did a parent or other adult in the household often or very often...
swear at you, insult you, put you down, or humiliate you? Or act in
a way that made you afraid that you might be physically hurt?

Did a parent or other adult in the household often or very often...
push, grab, slap, or throw something at you? Or ever struck you
that you had marks or were injured?

Did an adult or person at least five years older than you ever...
touch or fondle you or have you touch their body in a sexual way?
Or attempt or actually have oral, anal, or vaginal intercourse
with you?

Did you often or very often feel that... no one in your family loved
you or thought you were important or special? Or your family
didn't look out for each other, feel close to each other, or support
each other?

Did you often or very often feel that... you didn't have enough to
eat, had to wear dirty clothes, and had no one to protect you?
Or your parents were too drunk or high to take care of you or
take you to the doctor if you needed it?

Was a biological parent ever lost to you through divorce,
abandonment, or other reasons?

Was your mother or stepmother often or very often pushed,
grabbed, slapped, or had something thrown at her?
Or sometimes, often, or very often kicked, bitten, hit with a fist, or
hit with something hard? Or ever repeatedly hit or threatened
with a gun or knife?

Did you live with anyone who was a problem drinker or alcoholic,
or who used street drugs?

Was a household member depressed or mentally ill, or did a
household member attempt suicide?

Did a household member go to prison?

                                        Total Number of Y=

Tallying your ACE score is straightforward. The number of yes answers is your score. What does that number mean? It means a lot. Think of your score as a cholesterol reading for childhood toxic stress load.

The higher your ACE score, the higher your risk of health and social problems.

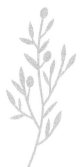

The higher your ACE score, the higher your risk of health and social problems.

With an ACE score of 4 or more, things start getting serious. Having a 4 or greater increases a person's risk of emphysema or chronic bronchitis by 400 percent and suicide risk by 1,200 percent.[34,35] Among other troubling tendencies, the likelihood of dealing with depressive episodes spikes to 460 percent. The risk of developing chronic pulmonary lung disease increases to 390 percent, and hepatitis risk goes to 240 percent.[36,37]

This graphic shows how the risk for unfavorable outcomes is tied to the number of ACEs a person has and areas where ACEs can have the most lasting effects:

ACES CAN HAVE LASTING EFFECTS ON...

 Health (obesity, diabetes, depression, suicide attempts, STDs, heart disease, cancer, stroke, COPD, broken bones)

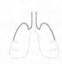 **Behaviors** (smoking, alcoholism, drug use)

 Life Potential (graduation rates, academic achievement, lost time from work)

Risk for Negative Health & Well-being Outcomes

ACES have been found to have a graded dose-response relationship with 40+ outcomes to date.

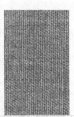

# of ACEs   1   2   3   4   ≥5

This pattern holds for the 40+ outcomes, but the exact risk values vary depending on the outcome

There are numerous other childhood traumas that the test doesn't take into account. These include bullying, racism, death of a loved one, serious injury, car accidents, being in the foster care system, homelessness, and much more. Your ACE score, therefore, does not tell the whole story but is meant more as a guideline and a predictor tool for future events and health outcomes.

Analysis of the ACE Study showed that higher levels of childhood mistreatment and lack of emotional support correlated with "significant and sustained losses" in health-related quality of life.[38,39] Here are some other disturbing statistics tied to the occurrence of one or more ACEs:

* **Autoimmune Disease.** Researchers showed that childhood traumatic stress increased the likelihood of hospitalization due to a diagnosed autoimmune disease in adulthood.[40]

* **Cancer.** Multiple human studies have identified significant associations between early adversity and cancer risk factors.[41] They concluded that childhood adversity in many forms may increase a person's cancer risk.[42,43,44]

* **Chronic Obstructive Pulmonary Disease (COPD).** Data from 26,546 adult women and 19,015 adult men in five states indicates that ACEs are related to COPD risk, especially among women.[45]

* **Frequent Headaches.** Researchers who examined the ACE Study results reported that the number of ACEs showed a graded relationship to frequent headaches in adults.[46]

* **Ischemic Heart Disease.** Scholars found a link between the number of ACEs and a person's risk of developing ischemic heart disease (IHD). They also suggested that psychological factors may be more significant than traditional risk factors in connecting ACEs to the development of IHD.[47]

* **Liver Disease.** The CDC determined that the number of ACEs correlates with liver disease. Compared with people with no ACEs, those with 6 or more have a 260 percent higher chance of having liver disease.[48]

• **Depression.** ACEs such as neglect and abuse have been identified as significant risk factors for adult depression and lower overall mental health scores.[49,50] In a test group of over 2,000 men and women in Ireland, researchers found that "exposure to any ACE (versus none) was associated with almost three times the odds of depressive symptoms."[51] In a study of almost 10,000 people in California, results indicated that childhood emotional abuse of any kind increased the risk for lifetime depressive disorders by 270 percent in women and 250 percent in men.[52]

• **Suicide.** After studying the answers of the original ACE Study subjects, researchers established that having one or more ACE in any category increased the risk of attempted suicide by 200 to 500 percent.[53]

Your ACE score may also negatively affect you by causing you to engage in dangerous behaviors. This helps explain your ACE score's tremendous influence on health and disease risk. Here are some tendencies that increase in likelihood as your ACE number rises:

1. **You are more likely to become obese.** Physical abuse and verbal abuse were most strongly associated with an increased risk of excess body weight and obesity.[54]

2. **You are more likely to abuse alcohol.** Having one or more ACEs increases your odds of abusing alcohol as an adult.[55] Depending on whether one or both parents abused alcohol, you have a significantly higher chance of having multiple ACEs.[56]

3. **You are more likely to use tobacco.** Particularly among women, psychological distress was responsible for a significant portion of the link between ACEs and smoking (21 percent for emotional abuse, 16 percent for physical abuse, 15 percent for physical neglect, and 10 percent for parental separation or divorce).[57]

4. **You are more likely to use drugs.** Compared to those with an ACE score of 0, people with an ACE score of 5 or more were 40 percent more

likely to abuse prescription drugs.[58] Also, each ACE increased the likelihood of illicit drug use by 200 to 400 percent.[59]

Researchers also concluded higher ACE scores correspond to more significant work performance impairment and increased odds of premature death.[60,61,62] With higher ACE numbers also comes greater incidences of fetal death associated with adolescent pregnancy, increased promiscuity rate, more sexual risk behaviors in young women, higher STD rates among both men and women, and increased teen pregnancy rate.[63,64,65,66]

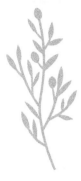

> **ACE scores could be *the* leading determinate of the health, social wellbeing, and the economy of the nation.**

From the data, it seems that ACE scores could be *the* leading determinate of the health, social wellbeing, and the economy of the nation.

For too long, we've been missing this in the pediatricians' offices and therapists' offices. It's time to make ACE testing a common occurrence in every kind of medical office in the country. I am now offering the ACE questionnaire in my office to all new patients. No matter how you look at it, the power wielded by the grownups who raised us is too strong to ignore.

Your Body is Keeping Score

Now that you know your ACE score, I'll tell you mine. It's 6. While it could absolutely be worse, it's not great, especially since a score of 4 or more is when the disease, depression, and mortality rates start to increase exponentially.

I have never been a partyer. I've never used illicit drugs or smoked, and I don't drink excessively. Still, because my score is 6, I have a higher risk of adverse health effects such as heart disease and cancer.

Also, unbeknownst to me, my body has been keeping track of the various forms of abuse I experienced. In the book, *The Body Keeps Score*, Bessel van der Kolk, MD, explains how childhood trauma has become America's most urgent and dire health crisis.[67]

Whether you realize it or not, your body is keeping a running tally of the trauma. For the multitude of people who have reported one or more ACEs, those experiences don't just magically fade away over time. Your body manifests trauma in some real way regardless of how long ago it was or whether or not you even remember it.

The saying "time heals all wounds" is simply not true.

But there is light at the end of the tunnel. Trauma *does* affect the whole person, but you are also a miracle of God with the ability to heal, repair, and rebuild. With intentional effort and refocusing, you can find peace and healing. You can also stop blaming yourself for things that were beyond your control.

> **The saying "time heals all wounds" is simply not true.**

I used to internalize the blame for all of my ACEs. Not anymore.

What happened to me when I was young wasn't my fault.

Do you know how long it took me to be able to say that and actually *mean* it? Most of my life. There are still some days that I momentarily revert back to that little girl who is desperately seeking approval. In those moments, I hurt physically and emotionally.

I'm not sure that pain will ever entirely go away, but I'm sure as heck not going to let that pain define me. I also see in retrospect that the way I was raised inadvertently propelled me to continue on and reach for more. I sought degree after degree in an attempt to hear my mom say just once, "I'm proud of you, Dani."

I never heard those words, and I never will, thanks to her deteriorating state of mental health, but it doesn't matter. I went down this path for a reason far more significant than my ego or desire for praise. I am here for my kids.

And I'm here for you.

With an ACE score of 6, the statistics say that I have a reduced lifespan of around 20 years.[68] The statistics also say that I am destined for depression and chronic disease. Well, I'm sorry, but I'm not going to accept that, and you don't have to accept what the numbers say either.

In statistics, there are these little things known as *outliers* that deviate from expectations and differ significantly from other observations.

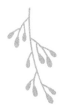

> **I'm proud to say that I'm an outlier.**

I'm proud to say that I'm an outlier.

You are stronger and more resilient than you know. You have everything in you right now to become an exception to the rules as well. If you'd like to join our tribe and become an outlier, just keep reading.

Flipping the Gene Switch

Adverse childhood experiences play an undeniably critical role in our outcomes as adults. That's the *nurture* side of the equation. Now, let's talk about the *nature* side of our health, also known as genetics.

Adults like to blame everything on our genes, from a lousy temperament and lack of patience to obesity and cancer. When something doesn't go right in our lives, our gut response is to blame forces outside of our control. High blood pressure, autoimmune disease, cancer, depression, pasta cravings, sugar addictions, and back seat driving—anything and everything gets thrown under the genetics umbrella.

I've been guilty of believing that my genetics would one day be my kryptonite. My grandmother had dementia, and now my mother has the disease. My mother attempted suicide as a teenager, and my maternal grandfather actually did die by suicide.

My mother also had postpartum *psychosis* after I was born and had to be institutionalized to recover. I was six weeks old, and she had stopped feeding me and didn't know daytime from nighttime. My dad was in the Navy and had to bring in help to care for me while mom was in a mental institution getting the help she needed to recover.

On paper, I'm a neural nightmare.

But I know something that my genes don't. I know that just because someone in my family had a disorder, that does not mean I will. Luckily, new science has emerged that gives us hope. It's called *epigenetics*, which is the study of changes in organisms that are caused by modification of gene expression rather than alteration of the genetic code itself.[69]

The Greek prefix *epi-* means "over, outside of, around." This implies bodily responses that are *in addition to* the traditional genetic basis for inheritance—or as I like to say, "beyond the DNA."

To better explain what I mean by "modification of gene expression" and why it matters, let's clarify a few terms. *Gene regulation* is how a cell controls which genes are "turned on" or expressed. *Gene expression* is what allows a cell to respond to its environment. It acts as an ON/OFF switch to control when proteins are made. Expression also acts as a volume control knob that increases or decreases the number of proteins made.

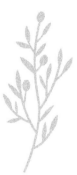

Epigenetics tells us that it's possible to wield some control over which genetic switches turn *on* and *off*.

In a nutshell, epigenetics tells us that it's possible to wield some control over which genetic switches turn *on* and *off*.

It's also important to note that a cell's gene expression pattern is determined by information from both inside *and* outside the cell. There's not much you can do to influence the information received from inside the cell, such as inherited proteins and DNA damage. However, you can absolutely control a portion of what affects a cell from the outside—and that zincludes food and environmental influences.

Arguably the most significant influencer on gene expression is nutrition. The human diet has undergone some serious changes over recent generations, and this trend is likely to keep right on going. The way most food is produced today is downright disgusting. Our internal monitoring systems don't even know how to handle the Frankenfoods grown in nutrient-depleted soil, produced through laboratory-engineered seeds, and obtained from antibiotic-riddled feedlot animals.

Epigenetics gives us clear evidence that diet and nutrition can directly influence the human genome.[70] And given the reversible nature of epigenetic information (aka the OFF switch), numerous studies highlight exciting opportunities to influence the aging process and disease progression.[71] Several important conclusions have emerged from these studies:[72,73]

- Rather than being entirely genetically predetermined, our life span appears to be largely *epigenetically* determined by outside influences.

- Diet and environmental influences can impact our life span by changing epigenetic information.

- Inhibitors of epigenetic enzymes (such as environmental influences and disease progression) heavily influence the life span of all living organisms.

In short, incorporating the six lifestyle habits in Part Two of this book is your best bet for putting the hypothetical gene expression ball in your court, thereby greatly influencing your overall health and life outcomes.

Could You Be an Outlier?

Although I was terrified that I would end up like my mother, I did not experience postpartum depression (or psychosis) after either of my children were born. Part of it could have been that those genes had not yet been expressed. I also believe that my mindset was a huge part of my victory over mental illness. I was determined not to go down the same path my mother did.

It wasn't until my marriage started crumbling that I felt compelled to take medication during that dark time in my life. Even then, I did everything I could to stop taking the antidepressants and only took them for a few years.

I was resolved to rise above and become an outlier.

If you are currently taking antidepressants or other prescription medications and trying to fight the good fight, you are not weak. I'm not shaming you, nor do I think you don't have the mental toughness it takes. We often need a life preserver when we are paddling through the deepest of waters.

Here is what I *am* also saying. Your mindset can make a remarkable difference—and thanks to neuroplasticity, it's never too late to retrain your brain to think differently.

When you want to change the way you eat, experts say you have to "retrain" your taste buds. It works the same for our minds. Renowned neuroscientist Dr. Michael Merzenich gave a TED Talk in 2004 called "Growing Evidence of Brain Plasticity." According to this brain research pioneer, the accepted idea that the adult brain is hard-wired and loses its ability to change after adolescence is not correct. Here is how Merzenich explains it in his book, *Soft-Wired: How the New Science of Brain Plasticity Can Change Your Life:*[74]

> "What recent research has shown is that under the right circumstances, the power of brain plasticity can help adults' minds grow. Although certain brain machinery tends to decline with age, there are steps people can take to tap into plasticity and reinvigorate that machinery."

Neuroplasticity describes brain changes that occur in response to experiences. If you had more than your fair share of ACEs growing up, the experiences that have shaped you thus far might have been overtly negative.[75] However, neuroplasticity tells us that that new *positive* experiences and favorable habits in adulthood can undo earlier programming.

Isn't that exciting?

The motto of the U.S. Army Corps of Engineers is, "The difficult we do today. The impossible takes a little longer." This was also the unspoken mantra of Galileo Galilei, Isaac Newton, Abraham Lincoln, Amelia Earhart, Mother Teresa, Martin Luther King Jr., and every other world-changer who ever lived.

Before Ferdinand Magellan did it, the world thought sailing the entire ocean was impossible.

Before Roger Bannister did it, no one thought a human being could run a mile in under four minutes.

Before Wilbur and Orville Wright did it, no one thought it was possible to fly.

Before Marie Curie discovered it, no one even knew about radioactivity.

If these incredible feats are possible, isn't it possible for you to rise above a statistic, to re-train your brain so that you talk, act, and feel differently?

Isn't it possible for *you* to become an outlier? Your answer will have a lot to do with the kind of mindset you have, so let's figure out what that is.

Growth Mindset vs. Fixed Mindset

According to research that spans four decades, there are two mindsets: growth and fixed. Figuring out which one you have is not difficult. If you love to try new things and push yourself into unknown territory, you more than likely identify as *growth-mindset* oriented. If you prefer to stick to what you know, you are a *fixed-mindset* oriented person.[76]

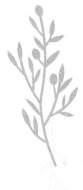

Growth-minded people simply believe that talent and triumph come through consistent effort, not through some mysterious birthright or genetics.

The theory behind these designations was developed by Stanford University psychologist Carol Dweck. She began studying the habits and attitudes of successful people to discover why some seem to thrive no matter what, while others struggle their entire lives in every area.[77]

Ironically, her research revealed that those who seem to be "naturals" in life are not natural-born successes at all.

Growth-minded people simply believe that talent and triumph come through consistent effort, not through some mysterious birthright or genetics.

Growth-minded individuals believe *anyone* can be the best at *anything*. Therefore, they know no limitations or boundaries. They succeed because they look at the achievements of others and think to themselves, "Hey, that could be me!" or just "Why not?" Therefore, they "naturally" develop enhanced capabilities through dedication, perseverance, and strategy.

For fixed mindsets, the future isn't so bright. According to them, intelligence, talent, and even health are things you have or do not have. They operate from an understanding that *inborn* talent and well-being ultimately determine success. If you don't have those at birth—well, that's too bad.

Add to a fixed mindset the deep-seated traumas caused by adverse childhood experiences, and you're in for a whole world of hurt.

Taking it a step further, if you have a fixed mind-set, research shows you are far more likely to give up. If you try a new sport and don't do well, for example, fixed mindsets will shrug their shoulders and say things like, "This isn't for me" or "I'm just not built for that."[78] Here is why this should matter to you:

> **The *Wild & Well* Way will only work if you believe you can change.**

The *Wild & Well Way* will only work if you believe you can change.

I want to transform your health and give you back your life, but it will require some radical alterations. There is a chance you could slip back into old behaviors as you begin to adjust your lifestyle habits.

Maybe that means you are too set in your ways to change. Or perhaps some people aren't meant to be healthy. Or maybe you're just one of those people who are genetically disposed to crave sugar and carbs, and there is nothing you can do about. Or possibly you were destined to be obese or have an autoimmune disease, and that's just your bad luck.

Don't believe these untruths!

You *can* do this, no matter your current habits, no matter how unwell you feel, no matter how much weight you need to lose, no matter how much pain or discomfort you are in today.

There is not a *single* person who is genetically predisposed to thrive on inflammatory, unhealthy foods. No one on this planet operates better when they are sleep deprived, sedentary, constipated, overstressed, and isolated. You have the opportunity every day to consciously make better choices. Adopting a growth mindset is essential for success and health. It's also the difference between a life full of excuses and regret and a life full of accomplishments, health, and joy.

Old habits and mindsets die hard. We all know this. But the key is that they can actually *die*.

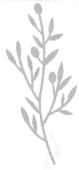

> **Old habits and mindsets die hard. We all know this. But the key is that they can actually *die*.**

You have the choice to seek growth. You can *choose* to believe that you won't suffer the way a family member has from a particular condition. You can *choose* to see your limitless potential.

However, you *also* have to desire health more than you desire the comfort of old habits or the ability to use genetics as an excuse for giving up.

Let's do a quick appraisal of your readiness to shift into a growth mindset and change old habits. Answer true or false to the following statements:

1. No matter who you are, you cannot significantly change your intelligence level.

   TRUE   **FALSE**

2. If I have to work really hard at something, it means I'm not naturally gifted.

   TRUE   **FALSE**

3. I do not enjoy trying difficult things.

   TRUE   **FALSE**

4. There are just some things I'll never be good at.

   TRUE   **FALSE**

5. People are born with a low, medium, or high level of intelligence, and that cannot change.

   TRUE   **FALSE**

6. When I do something incorrectly, I am not eager to try it again.

   TRUE   **FALSE**

The more "true" responses you gave, the more of a fixed mindset you have. One of my goals is to help you understand that you already have everything you need inside of you to overcome your diagnosis and find balanced health. But before we can get you there, you must fix in your mind that you will not fail and determine that you will succeed.

- If you are prone to speak words of negativity, commit to speaking words of life.

- If you are prone to looking at yourself in the mirror and feeling shame, commit to staring back at your reflection, and praising one of your many beautiful qualities.

- If you are prone to assuming the worst and writing your poor health off as an inevitability, commit to becoming an outlier.

I can't help you unless you are ready to fight. I'm like your preacher. His job is to give you the seeds to plant to live a better life, but what you do with those seeds once you step outside the church is up to you.

There is no reason to continue reading unless you commit to making changes. It does not matter what those changes are—just commit now.

Do You Deserve to Feel Better?

You may feel motivated as you are reading this book, but what happens the next time you are at a restaurant and the menu comes? What happens when the alarm goes off at 5:00 a.m. to head to the gym? What happens when you look in the mirror and see tired, baggy eyes? What happens when you walk down the grocery aisle? What happens when you are too exhausted from being a human taxi to fix dinner?

Your current state of health took you decades to reach. Naturally, you won't heal in ten days. Everybody wants instant results, and when they don't get them, they're quickly discouraged. If you are looking for immediate results, look elsewhere. The first step in the long road ahead is to *prove* to yourself that you deserve to be well—and you do that by putting your health at the top of your priority list.

If a pediatrician told you that the choices you were making for your children were killing them, you would alter those choices *immediately*.

How is it any different for your own body? Damaging lifestyle habits are killing you; if you want to live a longer life with more joy and less pain, you must stop.

Are you worth it?

You bet you are.

If you are angry like I was for so many years at the "unfair" hand I got dealt in my youth, it's time to take steps to heal. Consider finding a professional therapist who can help you dig in and let things go that are weighing down both your body and soul. Resentment is a powerfully destructive force, whether you feel it for your parents, your spouse, or yourself. Resentment causes you to stay stuck in the past, but here's the truth:

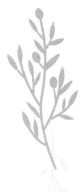

> **You are not your past. Commit to becoming a *visionary* who sees what could be, not a *historian* who only sees what once was.**

You are not your past. Commit to becoming a *visionary* who sees what could be, not a *historian* who only sees what once was.

You may be broken, and medication may be holding you together, but those wounds are too deep for Band-Aids over the long term. You were not designed to stay broken, but it is going to require you to dig to the root to fix the sources of the problem—not the tangible symptoms, but the intangible sources.

So, let me ask you again—are you worth it?

Do you believe your body can heal itself, and you can live a healthy and vibrant life? If you think it can be done, then you will find a way to make it a reality, because it *is* possible.

However, if you *don't* believe this can be your reality, then you are *also* right.

That's how powerful the mind is. Napoleon Hill said, "Whatever the mind can conceive and believe, it can achieve."

Start planting mental seeds of victory in the area of health. Trust your body. Trust your instincts. Then, determine to overcome the lie that your future is pre-determined by genetics or your upbringing and become the exception to the rule—the outlier—because it *is* possible.

Autoimmune disease is a bodily response, not a genetic inevitability. Obesity is almost always because of poor food choices. There are foods and environmental influences linked to the formation of every major disease. Inputs that outweigh genetics have caused your body to respond negatively.

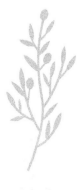

Change the input, both physically and mentally, and you can change those responses to better ones.

Change the input, both physically and mentally, and you can change those responses to better ones.

Do you want to heal your body? What will it feel and look like when you do? Will you be able to run a mile without stopping? Will you live to see your grandchildren get married? Whatever "victory" looks like to you, don't just speak it or think it, but play it out in your mind. What will people say when you tell them that you no longer take medication or that you just ran your first marathon? How will it feel to go back to the doctor 20, 30, or more pounds lighter?

Using descriptive terms, write out what it will look like to achieve your most significant health goal. When you're free from the limitations of an unwell body, here is how you will look and feel, and here is how other people will react:

_____

_____

_____

_____

_____

First thing in the morning, hit the play button in your mind on this visualization, and watch yourself achieving victory. This doesn't have to be a time-consuming activity. Do it while you are in the shower or brushing your teeth.

Decide to take the time for yourself.

In the wake of the horrible reality of the ACE study findings, researchers were desperate to discover protective factors that could mitigate the long-term impact of adverse childhood experiences.

Resiliency is the term they began using—and it's the ability to adapt well or "bounce back" in the presence of challenging life events. Having healthy, stable relationships and using established support systems are two ways to boost your resilience. No matter whether your ACE score is 0 or it's off the charts, strategies and resources exist to support you. We will discuss the power and importance of community later in the book.

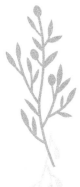

> **You can break the cycle of childhood trauma and step out of the shadow of your past.**

We are a broken society that is raising broken children, and, tragically, hurt people hurt *other* people. But take heart:

You *can* break the cycle of childhood trauma and step out of the shadow of your past.

You can build resilience through having relationships with those who love and support you. Find people who see your strengths, weaknesses, and scars… and love you for all of it. Seek out people who recognize your beautiful spirit and want to help you find your inner warrior and fight for the life God intended for you.

Jeremiah 29:11 tells us the *real* truth, "For I know the plans I have for you," declares the Lord, "plans to prosper you and not to harm you, plans to give you hope and a future."

You are *not* your past—but to break the cycle, you need to put on your oxygen mask first. It's time to learn how to take care of yourself so you can care for others. Stop blaming yourself, stop blaming genetics, and feel empowered through the knowledge that the damage inflicted by past traumas doesn't have to define you anymore.

wild & well Rx

Dani Williamson, MSN, FNP

R_x

Patient Name: ....

Age: .... Date: ....

1. Remember that your past does not have to predict your future.

2. Be the one to break the cycle of dysfunction in your family.

3. Find a therapist, counselor, or psychiatrist (there are sliding scale organizations all over the world) that will help you work through your past traumas.

4. Treat both your mental health and your physical health, because you can't have one without the other.

5. Write down your health goals and stick to them.

6. Remember that there was only ONE perfect human, and it's not you or me!

7. Tell your story because there is power in it! Write it out, speak it and know that you story is what makes you… you.

8. Create a vision board. Vision boards are powerful and help you visualize your ideal future.

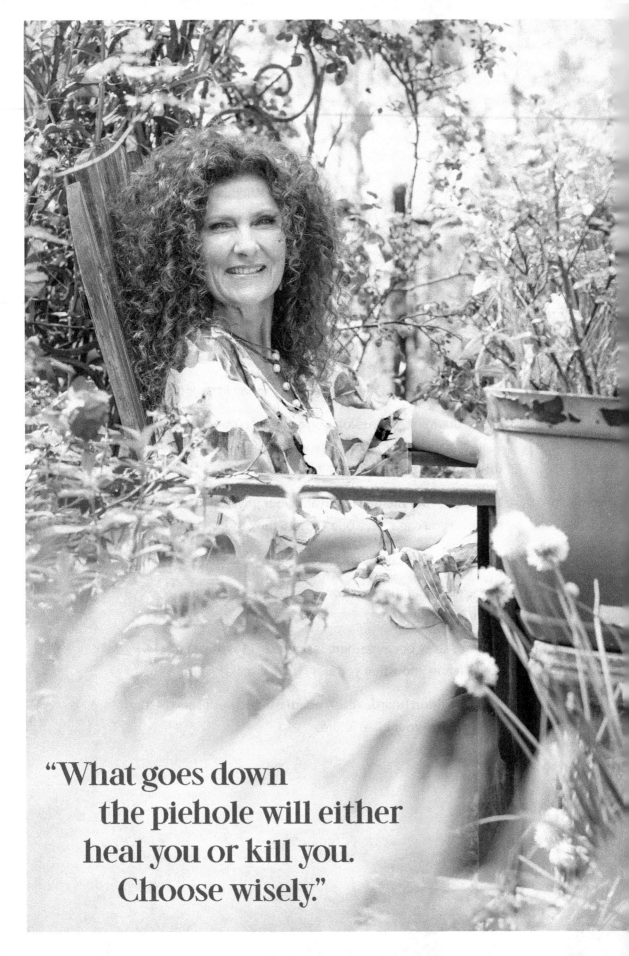

"What goes down the piehole will either heal you or kill you. Choose wisely."

inflammation
is the devil

*"The devil has put a penalty on all things we enjoy in life.
Either we suffer in our health, or we suffer in our soul, or we get fat."*

ALBERT EINSTEIN

If you are an adult with a TV and a smartphone, you've heard about inflammation. From Dr. Oz to the evening news, it's as much of a buzzword in the health headlines as *GMO*, *ketogenic*, and *good fats*.

What you may not know is that there are two kinds. *Acute inflammation* is what happens when you cut your finger, sprain your ankle, or catch the flu. Your body responds by sending white blood cells to help the injured area or area under attack from foreign invaders. You feel that telltale swelling and heat that lets you know your body is on the job.

Chronic inflammation is something else entirely. It's a slow, simmering immune response that never entirely goes away. Chronic inflammation is associated with fatigue, insomnia, anxiety, depression, cancer, chronic diseases, autoimmune disorders, neurodegenerative conditions, and more.[79,80,81]

The dictionary definition you see here only covers acute inflammation:

Inflammation [inflə' māSH(ə)n]

(*noun*): A local response to cellular injury that is marked by capillary dilatation, leukocytic infiltration, redness, heat, pain, swelling, and often a loss of function and that serves as a mechanism initiating the elimination of noxious agents and of damaged tissue.

That doesn't tell the whole story. It also doesn't do much to explain the kind of inflammation that can simmer for decades before you begin to see or—probably more accurately—*recognize* symptoms. Here is my definition that better explains chronic inflammation:

Dani's Definition of Inflammation [inflə' māSH(ə)n]

(*noun*): Your body's response to poor diet, lack of exercise, inadequate sleep, chronic bowel issues, insufficient stress management, and lack of community connection. You may have no symptoms until you develop a disease, or you may experience symptoms from the start. Treating symptoms will not make it go away and, in many cases, will only make things worse.

Chronic inflammation slowly festers until it manifests as fatigue, body aches, itching, dry eyes, shortness of breath, insomnia, weight gain, and decreased libido. There are so many symptoms of chronic inflammation that it might be easier to list what's *not* a symptom. As one example, postnasal drip is a commonly missed inflammation indicator. That simple little sniff and nighttime congestion are not so harmless. Such symptoms are blatant signs of chronic inflammation that are often linked to food sensitivities (more on that in Chapter Five).

More significantly, research ties chronic inflammation to many of the diseases on the rise around the world. These include but are not limited to cancer, depression, type 2 diabetes, obesity, and autoimmune diseases such as rheumatoid arthritis and Hashimoto's thyroiditis.[82,83,84,85]

Have you ever wondered why so many painful conditions end with "itis?" There is an excellent reason for that. The suffix "itis" literally means inflammation. There is chronic inflammation behind the development of each condition, from arthritis, gastritis, and colitis to sinusitis, thyroiditis, and vasculitis.

For many people, it can be challenging to determine which is causing which. In other words, is it the chronic inflammation that's causing the disease, or is it the disease that's causing the inflammation? This is the puzzle that I work to solve every day, and it's what functional medicine is designed to do—to discover what's causing that "itis." That is why we are going to spend the remaining sections in this chapter answering some common questions about inflammation.

What Signals the Body to Become Inflamed?

Before we address what causes your body to have inflammatory responses and discuss how to decrease inflammation, we need to talk about cytokines. *Cytokines* are small proteins secreted by the immune system that are designed to protect you when your body is under attack. They signal to your cells that something is affecting the body's perfect balance, and you need help.[86]

There are pro-inflammatory cytokines that increase inflammation, and there are anti-inflammatory cytokines that calm inflammation. In some cases, this marvelous defense system does its job flawlessly and restores balance in the body. Other times, however, the overproduction of cytokines may actually do more harm than good.[87] When there are too many pro-inflammatory cytokines, you are going to have problems—lots of problems:

* **Pain.** Significant evidence links certain cytokines to the presence of chronic pain.[88]

* **Chronic Stress.** If you are overstressed and overworked, your body is in a constant immunosuppressive state.[89] The body overproduces the pro-inflammatory cytokines to address the constant immune stress.[90] That means that your stress is literally killing you by producing substances linked with an array of deadly conditions.[91]

- **Depression.** If you suffer from depression, cytokine-induced inflammation may also be to blame. Studies of depressed patients show a high level of proinflammatory cytokines.[92]

- **Obesity.** A study found that the high levels of pro-inflammatory cytokines present in obese, type 2 diabetics relate mainly to their obesity rather than to their type 2 diabetes. In other words, the adipose tissue (body fat) is what is causing the most significant inflammatory response.[93]

- **Cognitive Decline.** Science has connected elevated cytokine levels to an increased risk of conversion from mild cognitive decline to Alzheimer's disease. An imbalance between pro-inflammatory and anti-inflammatory cytokines has even been linked to other neurological conditions such as bipolar disorder.[94]

- **Autoimmune Disease.** Specific cytokines known as CD4+ T helper cells are critical for proper immune cell homeostasis and host defense. Unfortunately, they are also primary contributors to the pathology of auto-immune diseases.[95]

- **Heart Failure.** Pro-inflammatory cytokines are positively linked to the development and progression of heart failure.[96]

- **Cancer.** Some cytokines are designed to slow tumor growth. Unfortunately, pro-inflammatory cytokines can promote cancer growth and facilitate cell invasion and metastatic growth.[97]

When your body perceives a threat to homeostasis (total body balance), it is going to react. There is nothing you can do to stop your immune system from producing cytokines in response to adverse food choices, stress, or other environmental toxins. You can't eat a donut and tell your body to pretend that it's broccoli. What you *can* do is stop giving it a reason to produce pro-inflammatory cytokines by making better choices.

What Are Some Hidden Causes of Inflammation?

Research shows that inflammation can begin from the moment we're born or even before.[98,99] Studies indicate that newborn babies who have decreased amounts of certain gut bacteria have an increased risk for inflammatory reactions such as seasonal allergies, food sensitivities, and food allergies.[100] Studies have also shown that processed foods, lack of sleep, excess stress, poor gut health, and low-grade viral infections (such as Epstein-Barr, herpes simplex, and the chickenpox virus) all contribute to chronic inflammation.[101,102] Genetics and other factors beyond our control play a part in disease development. However:

The majority of conditions we face today are a direct result of toxic accumulation that leads to inflammation and, eventually, disease.

God designed our bodies to defend against toxicity, but the human body has its limits. Common signs of toxic overload include:[103]

> **The majority of conditions we face today are the direct result of toxic accumulation that leads to inflammation and, eventually, disease.**

- Gradual cognitive decline

- GI issues such as bad breath, constipation, bloating, and gas

- Headaches, fatigue, body aches, and pains

- Stubborn belly fat

- Skin problems

- Food cravings, especially for sugar and processed foods

- Irritability and mood swings

Maybe you eat "clean" and take other active steps to limit your exposure to excess toxins. If so, then you are on the right track. For many of my patients, however, they are shocked at how insidious toxins are in their daily lives. In short, toxins are everywhere.

The six lifestyle areas in this book have the most significant effect on toxicity and inflammation levels. If there can only be one primary culprit, however, I'd choose eating habits every time.

The Standard American Diet (commonly called the SAD diet) is filled with precisely what you think it is: processed, packaged, bagged, canned, tubed fake foods. It is high in carbs, sugar, inflammatory fat, and nutritionally-devoid protein. The SAD diet includes all of America's favorite meals and snacks—from the gas station and the fast-food drive-through to the buttery, genetically modified popcorn at the movies and the cake at your kid's birthday party.

We will address foods that are common parts of the SAD diet in Part Two, so get ready. We will also discuss the anti-inflammatory effects of getting adequate sleep, balancing your gut, exercising, reducing stress, and finding your tribe. For this section, though, let's focus on hidden and environmental factors that are affecting your body in negative ways and causing chronic inflammation.

Environment. Chemicals are everywhere. They are in your food, the air, and the environment all around you. Do you smoke or live with a smoker? Do you eat conventionally grown foods that are laced with pesticides and fertilizers? Do you live near chemical plants? I grew up in a town where chemical plants lined the river, and I don't believe it is a coincidence that my hometown has a higher-than-average cancer rate.

> **Chemicals in the environment are going to find their way into your body and hurt you. This is not groundbreaking news.**

Chemicals in the environment are going to find their way into your body and hurt you. This is not groundbreaking news.

A 1984 study published in *Environmental Health Perspectives* found that residential exposure to petroleum and chemical air emissions is linked to increased rates of oral, throat, stomach, lung, prostate, kidney, and urinary cancers. Researchers also discovered a strong tie between residential chemical exposure and mortality rates of cardiovascular disease and cirrhosis of the liver.[104]

The household cleaners you use and the new paint you just bought for the remodel are also riddled with chemicals. Just because something dries doesn't mean you can no longer absorb its chemical ingredients through your skin or inhale them. Dermatitis (notice the "itis") is the most widely recognized effect of everyday household product use.[105] Respiratory tract inflammation and damage, including the development of asthma, are also linked to the chemicals in household products and mainstream commercial paints that contain volatile organic compounds (VOCs).[106,107]

There are alternative cleaning products available that use essential oils as their active ingredients. Don't forget good old-fashioned vinegar! Vinegar is just as effective as commercial cleaners at disinfecting surfaces in laboratory studies.[108] Save money and your health by making your own household cleaners. This includes laundry detergents, carpet shampoos, and air fresheners. Stop washing your clothes in inflammatory chemicals and spraying them all over your house!

Water Supply. The water you drink and the water you use to bathe and cook also matter. The U.S. Department of Agriculture has estimated that 50 million people in this country obtain their drinking water from sources that are potentially contaminated by pesticides and other agricultural chemicals.[109] In one study, children ages three to six showed notable levels of pesticide exposure—not just from their food, but also from their water supply and their environment (even the carpet).[110]

Municipal water supplies are not fit to drink. If you haven't already, switch to distilled, reverse osmosis, or spring water. Also, consider a whole-house water filtration system. Filtering the water supply in your home can be pricey. Still, it won't be as expensive as the medical bills for treating diseases such as bladder cancer, which has been linked to long-term tap water use and consumption.[111]

Personal Care Products. Do you use drugstore hair, face, and body products? I'm talking about cosmetics, lotions, makeup, shampoo, conditioner, hair color, styling products, lipstick, nail polish, and nail polish remover. The environmental toxins contained within most major brands contribute to the toxic load in the body.

Sodium lauryl sulfate, a surfactant used in the majority of shampoos, soaps, and body washes, is linked to the production of pro-inflammatory cytokines that cause skin irritation and acute inflammation.[112] It stands to reason, then, if you use the products daily, the acute inflammation will eventually become chronic inflammation.

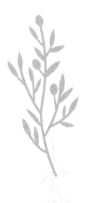

In cosmetics alone, the European Union has banned more than 1,300 chemicals. The United States? Only 11 chemicals have been outlawed.

The fragrances in perfume, cologne, shampoo, deodorant, and lotion contain synthetic chemicals that have been linked to allergies, reproductive toxicity, and even cancer.[113] Research published in *Environmental Health Perspectives* indicates that fragrance products contain more than 100 volatile organic compounds, including some that are classified as toxic or hazardous by federal law.[114]

Our country is far behind Europe in banning many of the hazardous chemicals found in so many of our products. In 2019, a proposed bill put forth by the Connecticut legislation called for cosmetics in their state to "meet the chemical safety standards established by the European Union."[115]

In cosmetics alone, the European Union has banned more than 1,300 chemicals. The United States? Only 11 chemicals have been outlawed.

Don't wait for adverse health problems to surface and laws to be written before you start reading ingredients labels and being more careful about what you put on your body.

Oral Health. The heath of your mouth, gums, and teeth are also a considerable part of the inflammation picture. A study published in the *Journal of Clinical Periodontology* concluded that there is a positive correlation between poor oral health and chronic inflammation that leads to coronary heart disease.[116] If you haven't been to the dentist in a while, it's time to go. Don't wait until you have to visit because you are in pain or experiencing discomfort. When it comes to your teeth, a proactive approach is the only approach that works.

Adipose Tissue. Mounting evidence highlights the role of adipose tissue (body fat) in the development of chronic inflammation that contributes to vasculopathy and cardiovascular risk.[117] Adipose tissue plays such a tremendous role in our health that it is now classified as an "organ" that interacts in immune and endocrine system functions! Adipose tissue releases numerous components that are shown to cause both inflammation and insulin resistance.[118,119]

When it comes to losing fat, it should never be all about the scale. There are far better indicators of healthy fat loss, and they are the diagnostic criteria for metabolic syndrome, as shown in this table. If you want to track a measurement, why not track waist circumference? It's a far better measure of your overall health and disease risk.

DIAGNOSTIC CRITERIA FOR METABOLIC SYNDROME*

Criterion	Definition
Abdominal obesity	Waist circumference: men, >40in. (>102cm); women, >35in. (>88cm)
Hypertriglyceridemia	≥150 mg/dL
Low HDL-C	Men, >40mg/dL; women, >50mg/dL
High blood pressure	≥130/85 mmHg
High fasting glucose	110/85 mg/dL

*Diagnosis based on presence of three of five factors.

Antibiotics. Excessive antibiotic use is a significant problem in this country. We hear regular news reports about the antibiotic-resistant strains that have developed thanks to the lazy way medical professionals treat virtually everything.[120] Doctors are becoming more careful to prescribe antibiotics only when necessary (and no longer in response to every sniffle that is probably caused by a virus anyway).

However, the doctor's office isn't even the most significant problem anymore. Approximately 80 percent of antibiotic use in the U.S. is in livestock, according to estimates based on the FDA's data on sales of antibiotics by manufacturers for food-producing animals.[121]

> I tell patients every day, "You're only as healthy as the animals you're eating."

To me, that is a terrifying statistic.

If you and your family are eating fast food and your kids are eating school lunches, you are eating toxic meat that is filled with not only antibiotics but also hormones and pesticides. It's no wonder why young women are developing more quickly than in the past and why more young men are developing breasts.[122,123]

Scientists in Europe have proven that restricting the use of antimicrobial agents in animals decreases antimicrobial resistance in humans—and that's without compromising animal health or significantly increasing the cost of food production.[124] Since antibiotic use is pervasive in the U.S., the only way to know for sure that the product is antibiotic-free is to buy organic. "USDA Organic" is a label protected and regulated by the U.S. Department of Agriculture.

I tell patients every day, "You're only as healthy as the animals you're eating."

Other Drugs. Non-steroidal, anti-inflammatory drugs (NSAIDs) that include ibuprofen and acetaminophen are chemical agents designed to decrease inflammation. While they are effective at calming *acute* inflammation, they could increase *chronic* inflammation and play a contributing role in the development of inflammatory bowel disease.[125,126] Oral birth control has been linked to inflammation and the development of conditions such as Crohn's disease and breast cancer.[127,128] Proton pump inhibitors that decrease stomach acid have been shown to increase inflammation and are associated with dementia and Alzheimer's.[129]

Modern life does not make it easy on our bodies. The systems and organs designed to keep us healthy and free of disease are being brutally assaulted daily. The air we breathe, the water we drink, the products we use, the foods we eat, the pills we take, and the stress we experience all appear to be working to destroy any chance of a vibrant, healthy life.

There doesn't seem to be much about modern life that is good for us. While it is harder to escape toxins, it is *still* possible when you are armed with knowledge and the burning desire to feel better!

Is Inflammation Reversible?

Your body is a self-healing organism and a truly remarkable machine. It makes lemonade out of lemons. Every. Single. Day. When you feed it pure junk, it still functions for you. It does an incredible job—until one day it doesn't. The body can only take so much. Eventually, when it's out of balance and inflamed for long enough, things start to malfunction.

The good news is unless you are dead, there is room for improvement.

When it comes to reversing inflammation, the only option for long-term success is a functional approach. Functional or integrative medicine practitioners pay close attention to all potential contributors to health and disease, including ACE testing, genetics, and environmental and lifestyle factors.

> **The good news is unless you are dead, there is room for improvement.**

With functional medicine, the goal is to address the whole person and the underlying causes of symptoms instead of making an isolated diagnosis based on what patients say they "feel" like. My doctors treated me based on how I *felt* on any given day, and the end result was over two decades of pure agony.

My practice is a blend of functional and modern medicine. I integrate conventional methods and the use of diagnostic techniques such as lab testing. Then I take it a step further by focusing on prevention through nutrition, exercise, gut health, stress management, and community connection. I also use a variety of treatments that include synthetic drugs and botanical medicines, therapeutic diets, supplements, stress-management techniques, and other natural therapies.[130]

When you come to my office, we don't start with your weight, blood pressure, and apparent symptoms. I dig, and then I keep digging. What do you eat? Do you keep a food log? How often do you exercise? What are your bowel movements like? Do you watch TV before bed or scroll through Facebook? Do you feel stressed? Are you and your spouse having sex anymore? Do you feel isolated from or connected with others?

That's the beginning.

I also want to know about your childhood and earlier years:

- Did you feel well when you were growing up?

- What was your home life like?

- Are you fully immunized?

- Have you ever had mono or chickenpox?

- Did you or do you live in a home with lead paint or copper pipes?

- Do you have mercury amalgams in your mouth?

- Have they been removed?

- Do you currently or have ever lived in a home with mold exposure?

- Were you abused as a child? Are you ; currently?

- Do you have breast implants?

What about family history? As we discussed in the previous chapter, genetics are a part of the picture, but it's only a fraction of the story. Just because your mother has diabetes, your grandfather died of heart disease, or your father struggles with migraine headaches doesn't mean you will. Remember, you are not your past *or* your family's past. Dementia may "run in my family," but I will do everything in my power not to express those genes. If I do get dementia, it won't be because drank diet sodas for decades, ate the SAD diet, smoked since I was 12, never exercised, and didn't get enough sleep. [131,132,133,134,135]

With women, we talk about their personal care routine. The average woman comes into contact with 168 chemicals before we ever walk out of the bathroom in the morning. [136] What about birth control and feminine product use? Grocery store tampons and pads contain pesticide-ridden cotton! If you're using traditional feminine products, you're pumping needless chemicals into your bloodstream.

Often, before patients ever leave the appointment, we've already focused in on the key factors that are likely contributing to their symptoms. When we address these factors, the first response that my patients usually experience is a decrease in symptoms. What does that mean? Decreased inflammation!

Once you stop signaling to your body to put up its defenses, those pro-inflammatory cytokines get a much-needed vacation.

> **Once you stop signaling to your body to put up its defenses, those pro-inflammatory cytokines get a much-needed vacation.**

As inflammation decreases, other satisfying side effects start manifesting, such as memory improvement, mental sharpness, energy level spikes, better sleep, increased sex drive, and weight loss. It's exciting to watch patients decrease their inflammation by changing their diets, drinking cleaner water, getting better sleep, moving their bodies, and taking the right supplements. It's also humbling to watch as they start to enjoy life again.

This is not rocket science. I'm using a time-tested form of medicine, established information, and science to help you decrease inflammation. Functional medicine is not based on a "take this because I'm the expert" mentality. We partner with patients to educate them. You need to know WHY your body is not functioning correctly if you ever hope to feel better. You must learn how to turn down the inflammation by focusing on what's causing it in the first place.

Can a functional medicine practitioner guarantee you will be inflammation free? No—but one sure thing is that our bodies are designed to heal themselves. However, wishing and hoping to feel better is not a strategy. You need the right knowledge, and then you need to take action!

What Supplements Help Decrease Inflammation?

Here is my general rule about supplements: They are great for doing what their name suggests—to *supplement* the primary elements of a wellness plan. No number of pills, powders, or tinctures in the world can overcome a toxic diet and lifestyle.

I use food as the primary form of medicine. Still, if you are doing all the things right in the six lifestyle areas, a few essential supplements may enhance your results. There are four supplements I recommend most people take, no matter your state of health to help build a strong foundation for healing.

PROBIOTICS

A high-quality, shelf-stable probiotic is your partner in the fight to reduce inflammation.[137] Look for reputable brands such as MegaSpore and Master Supplements. Also, be sure to purchase a product with a higher number of probiotics, from 15 billion to 100 billion, and 10 to 30 different strains. Look for key strains such as spore-based *Bacillus coagulans*, *Saccharomyces boulardii*, *Bacillus subtilis*, *Lactobacillus rhamnosus*, and other cultures or formulas that ensure the probiotics make it to the gut and can colonize.

Your natural inclination, based on popular opinion, is to head straight to the refrigerated section of the health food store for probiotics. The problem with that is if those strains are so fragile that they can't handle being stored at room temperature, how are they going to handle your 98.6-degree stomach and stomach acid?

Be careful not to spend $50 or more on a probiotic that has no proof that it actually survives the journey from the mouth to the intestines. If you do that, the only benefit you'll receive is being able to say you have expensive poop. Do your homework and identify the strains that support your specific needs (ask a functional medicine practitioner for help if you are unsure). You can also eat probiotic-rich, fermented foods such as kimchi, kefir, natto, and kombucha.

MULTIVITAMIN

Your body has a complex microbiome that we will discuss in-depth in Part Two, and so does the earth's soil in which your food is grown and upon which animals graze.[138] Sadly, the earth's soil is not the same as it used to be. As a result, even the most nutritionally dense foods may not provide you with everything you need.

I recommend a whole-food-based, organically sourced multi such as Phytomulti Vitamin from Metagenics to supplement an already-healthy diet. That is the only vitamin I have used myself or in my office for the past eight years. It's the number one seller for Metagenics in their line of over 400 products for a reason—IT WORKS. Each daily serving contains seven to nine servings of fruits and vegetables and all of the methylated B vitamins essential for detoxification. We offer it in our supplement store and our online store.

FISH OIL

There are many quality fish oil supplements made from a variety of fish, with the most common ones being halibut, tuna, salmon, cod liver, mackerel, and herring. Fish oils contain omega-3 fatty acids, which are shown to exhibit anti-inflammatory and inflammation-resolving effects.[139] Another popular and potent source of DHA and EPA (omega-3 fatty acids) is krill oil.

Omega-3 oils supplements are commonly found in capsules or soft gels. The coating masks the fishy smell but can also cover up rancid oil. If you take omega-3 capsules, it may be a good idea to open one from time to time and smell it to make sure it hasn't gone rancid. I use the Metagenics and Nordic Naturals omega supplements in my store, but there are other quality brands as well. Read both labels and reviews for sourcing information.

VITAMIN D

It would be great if we all got an hour or more of direct sunlight every day. Your skin can naturally synthesize enough vitamin D through direct sunlight to enhance immune function, fight disease, improve mood, and help maintain a healthy weight.[140]

For most of us, however, that is just not feasible, which is why I recommend everyone take a high-quality vitamin D supplement. Look for one that contains vitamin D3, also known as cholecalciferol. Check the label and find one with minimal added ingredients or fillers. Keep in mind that vitamin D is a fat-soluble vitamin. If your vitamin D supplement doesn't contain oil, take it with a meal that includes a good source of fat (such as ghee, olive oil, or a slice of avocado) to optimize absorption.

Again, I rely on Metagenics and a few other brands for their D3 plus K2 in the office. Vitamin D3 needs K2 to improve absorption. Vitamins D3 and K2 are fat soluble vitamins, and I do not recommend starting these or continuing on them long-term without first knowing your nutrient levels.

If you do not have a primary care provider who can check labs for you, you can order labs online through Ulta Labs or other companies offering similar services.

It's important for you to know that I do not receive compensation from any supplement company to promote their products. I simply believe in the brands I choose because I trust their manufacturing processes and I've personally seen the results from their superior products.

There are several other supplements I recommend for decreasing inflammation:

* **Glutathione** is a master antioxidant—a powerful tool to fight the damaging effects of oxidative stress. You will read more about antioxidants and their oxidative stress- and disease-fighting powers in Chapter Four. I recommend a liposomal version that is designed to penetrate cells more quickly. Liposomes are like suitcases that can efficiently encapsulate materials and deliver them unharmed.[141]

* **Vitamin C** is also ideal for decreasing inflammation. I personally take 3,000 mg of ascorbic acid vitamin C every day. Vitamin C is water-soluble, and you aren't likely to overdose on it. You know you've taken too much when your stools become loose. If that happens, decrease your dosage.

* **Frankincense** and **lavender** oils are two of my all-time favorite essential oils for decreasing inflammation. Frankincense displays remarkable anti-inflammatory properties when used externally and, in some cases, internally.[142] (Consult with a medical professional before ingesting any essential oil.) Lavender essential oil is shown in laboratory studies to reduce localized swelling (edema) significantly.[143]

* **Turmeric** can significantly help reduce inflammation. Curcumin, the active ingredient in turmeric, is shown in scientific studies to diminish at least two key inflammatory markers (IL-6 and COX-2).[144] I take a turmeric supplement every day. Along with removing dairy from my diet, supplementing daily with turmeric has eliminated the joint pain I once experienced with lupus. I use a triple combination supplement with turmeric, frankincense, and xanthohumol from Metagenics.

Don't let anyone shame you into not taking a drug that helps you feel better in the short term. You may need a stopgap pharmaceutical option to get you through an acute phase. However, you also need a game plan for getting off that drug in the future. As you begin to heal, you will likely find that you need less and less medication.

I have an expensive education that taught me to identify conditions and treat their symptoms. I didn't learn to look for root causes until I learned functional medicine. There are underlying causes for your headache, heartburn, diarrhea, constipation, weight loss, weight gain, rash, insomnia, pain, autoimmune disease, anxiety, and depression. Functional medicine practitioners act as detectives, looking at ALL the clues and getting to the bottom of the mystery.

Pharmaceuticals have their place. I personally take low-dose naltrexone, which is for chronic inflammation and autoimmune disease. I take progesterone at night as well. For everything else, I "medicate" with a clean, green antioxidant diet and the healing lifestyle habits you will learn in this book.

How Badly Do You Want This?

The more stressed, over-scheduled, undernourished, unslept, sedentary, and isolated you are, the more inflammation you will have. Improper diet, lack of sleep, gut imbalance, high stress, inactivity, and lack of connection can turn on adverse responses. The good news is we also know what turns them back off again.

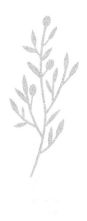

Improper diet, lack of sleep, gut imbalance, high stress, inactivity, and lack of connection can turn on adverse responses.

Change your diet, sleep habits, activity level, restroom patterns, stress level, and level of community connection, and you will look and feel better. You will also find the joy you thought would never return.

You will smile. You will love. You will heal.

You were not born with high blood pressure, type 2 diabetes, high cholesterol, or lupus. You were not born with depression, anxiety, rheumatoid arthritis, osteoarthritis, Hashimoto's thyroiditis, or insomnia. Those are innate, internal responses that an individual chooses to turn on or off through life style habits.

I'll repeat it: Your body is designed to heal. I haven't had IBS in ten years, and I don't itch anymore. I still have lupus, but 99 percent of the time, I'm symptom-free. I'm not depressed anymore, and I don't suffer from chronic anxiety. I am proof that the body is designed to repair itself, and that is what's so exciting about functional medicine.

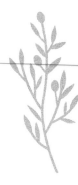

Find the root cause, and you could eliminate the need for medications that treat the symptoms!

What I practice is not just functional medicine, but **commonsense** medicine. Had only one doctor in 24 years ever asked, "Dani, what are you eating?"—my whole world would have changed. Imagine if one of my gastroenterologists had looked up from my colonoscopy results and said, "This doesn't make sense; let's talk about your home life and your diet." If one of them had, I don't believe I would have traveled down the road toward depression and autoimmune disease.

There are so many pieces to the puzzle that is your health.

If it were easy to be healthy, vibrant, and disease-free, the U.S. obesity rate wouldn't be rapidly approaching 40 percent, heart disease wouldn't be the number one killer in America, over 46 million people in the world wouldn't be suffering from dementia, and one of out every four Americans wouldn't be dying from cancer.[147,148,149,150]

Stop beating yourself up for "getting things wrong." If you aren't living your best life due to chronic inflammation, I want you to find hope in the truth that your body has a self-righting mechanism. You may only get one liver, one heart, two lungs, and so on, but unless your organs are entirely destroyed or removed, you have the chance to help heal and rebuild them!

An integrative, functional approach to addressing your health concerns requires a lot of work, but have you ever accomplished anything worthwhile without work? Think about these statements:

- "I could never get my family to eat like that."

- "I'm just a picky eater."

- "Natural products are too expensive."

- "I don't have time to work out."

When I hear one of these declarations, I know it's a patient who won't be with me for long. You've got to want it badly enough to make radical changes! You've got to want to be your best—for you, the Lord, your kids, your career, and your partner. If you don't have that desire, I can't do anything for you. So, let me ask you:

Are you tired of feeling tired?

Are you sick of feeling sick?

What are you going to do about it?

I hope your answer is "whatever it takes!"—and if it is, then I'm excited and honored to be a part of your Wild & Well journey.

wild & well Rx

Dani Williamson, MSN, FNP

℞ Patient Name: _____

Age: _____ Date: _____

1. Find a provider that works for you and addresses the full body. We work for you; you should fire us if we aren't doing our job!

2. Dig into what is causing your inflammation. Take note, be curious, and be alert to how you feel after eating, sleeping, etc.

3. Buy household brand that are less toxic as you run out of inflammation causing beauty products and cleaning supplies.

4. Don't be fooled by greenwashing. Do your homework (watch my YouTube videos on this at Dani Williamson Wellness) and thank me later.

5. Stop drinking out of plastic (glass is my favorite) and consider buying a water filter.

6. Take vitamins and make sure they good quality. Do not buy supplements on Amazon. There is no way to tell you are getting what you ordered!

7. Write down your medical history from birth. From antibiotic use, immunizations, molds, diet, and other toxic burdens to the environment in your hometown.

8. Ask yourself how sick and tired you are of being sick and tired. Your answer determines how committed you'll be.

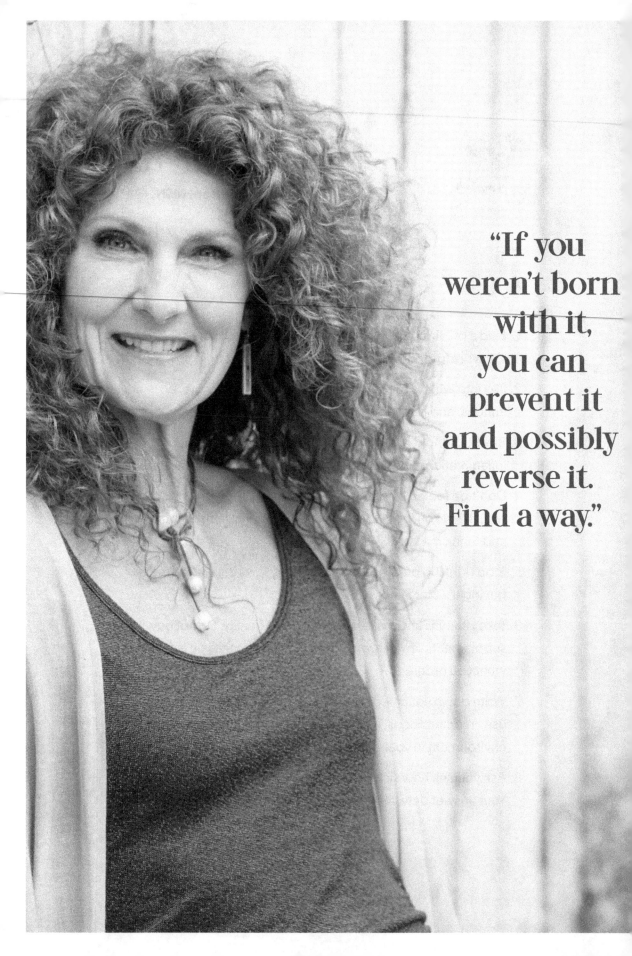

"If you weren't born with it, you can prevent it and possibly reverse it. Find a way."

disease from
sea to shining sea

"First, the doctor told me the good news.
I was going to have a disease named after me."
STEVE MARTIN

Life was once grueling and grim for the people of modern-day America. For the colonists during pre-Revolutionary-War times to the settlers who headed west during the 1800s expansion, every day was one big physical mountain to overcome.

If you were among the first to arrive in this land, the odds were not in your favor. Between 1607 and 1624, as many as 10,000 colonists arrived, but out of that number, only 1,275 survived.

From the time the sun came up until it set at night, men, women, and children worked their hands to the bone to forge a life for themselves, and, in many cases, to just stay alive.

Malaria, dysentery, and "winter illnesses" such as a cold and the flu were the top three killers during colonial times. These are known as endemic diseases that are localized and recur year after year. Endemic diseases such as malaria are terrifying. Unlike other illnesses such as measles and whooping cough that give you lifelong immunity after you've had them, you can catch malaria again—and again. The same goes for dysentery.

And, of course, no one only catches one cold or the flu in their lives and has lifelong immunity. Respiratory illnesses and all of their hundreds of strains and subtypes can return as often as they feel like it (you can even have two colds at the same time).

In a time when food was scarce, living conditions were unsanitary, and colonists were weakened by near-constant exposure to the elements, even the common cold could prove fatal.

Thanks to this reality, it was accepted that disease and premature death were part of life.

They were not living lives of luxury or ease by any stretch of the imagination.

Death in childbirth was common enough in colonial America for women to regard pregnancy with dread. In their letters, women often referred to childbirth as "the Dreaded apparition," "the greatest of earthly miseries," or "that evil hour I look forward to with dread." In a poem entitled "Before the Birth of One of Her Children," New England poet Anne Bradstreet wrote:

> How soon, my Dear, death may my steps attend,
> How soon't may be thy lot to lose thy friend.

In stark contrast, today, we write meticulous birth plans, create childbirth playlists on Spotify, and have gender reveal parties. We have the opportunity to celebrate life at every stage rather than dread what was once considered to be "the greatest of earthly miseries."

We live in a blessed time. If you have a roof, running water, electricity, and a refrigerator, you are truly living a life of opulence compared to the earliest pioneers of our great nation.

With access to modern medicine, widespread sanitization, hygiene practices, and knowledge of how the human body and immune system work,

Americans no longer live in fear of dying out in the fields of a mystery illness. Likewise, we are no longer forced to do backbreaking work or keep traveling in a covered wagon while a virus is running rampant in our bodies.

Today, our top three killers are something else entirely. Currently, the leading causes of death in America are cardiovascular disease, cancer, and unintentional injuries (including medical error).[151]

We are dying from two diseases that are clinically tied to lifestyle choices. We are also dying from errors made by medical professionals, mostly in the form of treatment and prescription error. And, since reporting that death is related to medical error is entirely voluntary, let's be honest: The wrongful death numbers are probably higher.

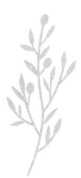

Had just ONE doctor asked me about my diet, my whole life would have been different.

Imagine what our ancestors would say if they knew that while they toiled away and barely had enough food to stay alive, we stuff our faces. Then we blindly put our trust in specialists who don't ask us what foods we're eating before they prescribe us the latest drug that their pharmaceutical rep has brought to the office for them to promote!

Had just ONE doctor asked me about my diet, my whole life would have been different.

Now, don't get me wrong. I'm incredibly thankful to be alive today. Grateful for modern medicine and scientific advancement. And I have no interest in returning to a time without toilets, hot showers, trauma surgery, or antibiotics.

However, I believe that with our great privileges and with the endless knowledge we now possess, we have a responsibility to do better.

We know that inflammation, environmental toxins, and stress affect disease formation. We also know that food is a crucial piece of the disease puzzle. So, I believe we owe it to ourselves and to our ancestors who died young in the pursuit of creating the greatest nation on Earth to make better choices.

But we all have to die of something, right?

It always burns me up when I hear that.

You live in America, which means you are free to live your life how you choose. For some, that means a diet of fast-food hamburgers, diabetes at 50 or younger, and a slow, steady decline in their health. For some, it means ignoring food sensitivities and known inflammatory agents such as pesticides and eventually developing autoimmune diseases and cancer.

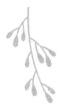

If you KNEW better, would you DO better?

But if you KNEW better, would you DO better?

I hope so—in fact, it's the entire premise for this book!

In this chapter, I will briefly cover today's most concerning disease trends. This is the last chapter that sets the stage for Part Two and the six pillars, so pay attention, and we'll move quickly.

The Autoimmune Epidemic

There is no shortage of alarming trends in modern society. Depending on your religious and political views, you are probably troubled about some politician, policy, or culture shift even as we speak.

No matter your views, there is one trend that should have everyone's attention—and that's the growing rates of autoimmune disease.

An autoimmune disease is a state in which your immune system mistakenly attacks your body. In an autoimmune disease, the immune system misidentifies part of your body, like your joints, skin, or thyroid gland as foreign. Some of the most commonly known autoimmune disorders are rheumatoid arthritis, lupus, inflammatory bowel diseases, psoriasis, type 1 diabetes mellitus, Hashimoto's thyroiditis, and psoriasis.

Autoimmune diseases are chronic and can be life-threatening, just as the rheumatologist told me decades ago when I was first diagnosed with lupus.

The National Institutes of Health (NIH) estimates that at least 24.5 million people have autoimmune disease in the U.S. On the other hand, the American Autoimmune Related Diseases Association (AARDA) says that the number is closer to 50 million Americans.

Why the disparity? The NIH numbers only included 24 diseases for which good epidemiology studies were available at that time.[152] Researchers have since identified 80 to 100 different autoimmune diseases and suspect at least 40 additional conditions of having an autoimmune origin.

The following is a list of the autoimmune conditions discovered so far. I don't expect you to read every single one of these diseases, but I'm including them here so you can understand the degree of this crisis (and by the time you are reading this, there may very well be even more added to this list):

Known Autoimmune Diseases

Achalasia	Autoimmune pancreatitis
Addison's disease	Autoimmune progesterone dermatitis (APD)
Adult Still's disease	Autoimmune retinopathy
Agammaglobulinemia	Autoimmune urticaria
Alopecia areata	Axonal & neuronal neuropathy (AMAN)
Amyloidosis	Baló disease
Ankylosing spondylitis	Behcet's disease
Anti-GBM/Anti-TBM nephritis	Benign mucosal pemphigoid
Antiphospholipid syndrome	Bullous pemphigoid
Autoimmune angioedema	Castleman disease (CD)
Autoimmune dysautonomia	Celiac disease
Autoimmune encephalomyelitis	Chagas disease
Autoimmune hepatitis	Chronic inflammatory demyelinating polyneuropathy (CIDP)
Autoimmune inner ear disease (AIED)	Chronic recurrent multifocal osteomyelitis (CRMO)
Autoimmune myocarditis	Churg-Strauss Syndrome (CSS) or Eosinophilic Granulomatosis (EGPA)
Autoimmune oophoritis	Cicatricial pemphigoid
Autoimmune orchitis	Cogan's syndrome

Known Autoimmune Diseases (cont.)

Cold agglutinin disease	Graves' disease
Congenital heart block	Guillain-Barre syndrome
Coxsackie myocarditis	Hashimoto's thyroiditis
CREST syndrome	Hemolytic anemia
Crohn's disease	Henoch-Schonlein purpura (HSP)
Dermatitis herpetiformis	Herpes gestationis or pemphigoid gestationis (PG)
Dermatomyositis	Hidradenitis Suppurativa (HS) (Acne Inversa)
Devic's disease (neuromyelitis optica)	Hypogammaglobulinemia
Discoid lupus	IgA Nephropathy
Dressler's syndrome	IgG4-related sclerosing disease
Endometriosis	Immune thrombocytopenic purpura (ITP)
Eosinophilic esophagitis (EoE)	Inclusion body myositis (IBM)
Eosinophilic fasciitis	Interstitial cystitis (IC)
Erythema nodosum	Juvenile arthritis
Essential mixed cryoglobulinemia	Juvenile diabetes (type 1 diabetes)
Bullous pemphigoid	Juvenile myositis (JM)
Evans syndrome	Kawasaki disease
Fibromyalgia	Lambert-Eaton syndrome
Fibrosing alveolitis	Leukocytoclastic vasculitis
Giant cell arteritis (temporal arteritis)	Lichen planus
Giant cell myocarditis	Lichen sclerosus
Glomerulonephritis	Ligneous conjunctivitis
Goodpasture's syndrome	Linear IgA disease (LAD)
Granulomatosis with Polyangiitis	Lupus

Known Autoimmune Diseases (cont.)

Lyme disease chronic	Peripheral neuropathy
Meniere's disease	Perivenous encephalomyelitis
Microscopic polyangiitis (MPA)	Pernicious anemia (PA)
Mixed connective tissue disease (MCTD)	POEMS syndrome
Mooren's ulcer	Polyarteritis nodosa
Mucha-Habermann disease	Polyglandular syndromes type I, II, III
Multifocal Motor Neuropathy (MMN) or MMNCB	Polymyalgia rheumatica
Multiple sclerosis	Polymyositis
Myasthenia gravis	Postmyocardial infarction syndrome
Myositis	Postpericardiotomy syndrome
Narcolepsy	Primary biliary cirrhosis
Neonatal Lupus	Primary sclerosing cholangitis
Neuromyelitis optica	Psoriasis
Neutropenia	Psoriatic arthritis
Ocular cicatricial pemphigoid	Pure red cell aplasia (PRCA)
Optic neuritis	Pyoderma gangrenosum
Palindromic rheumatism (PR)	Raynaud's phenomenon
PANDAS	Reactive Arthritis
Paraneoplastic cerebellar degeneration (PCD)	Reflex sympathetic dystrophy
Paroxysmal nocturnal hemoglobinuria (PNH)	Relapsing polychondritis
Parry Romberg syndrome	Restless legs syndrome (RLS)
Pars planitis (peripheral uveitis)	Retroperitoneal fibrosis
Parsonage-Turner syndrome	Rheumatic fever
Pemphigus	Rheumatoid arthritis

Known Autoimmune Diseases (cont.)	
Sarcoidosis	Temporal arteritis/Giant cell arteritis
Schmidt syndrome	Thrombocytopenic purpura (TTP)
Scleritis	Tolosa-Hunt syndrome (THS)
Scleroderma	Transverse myelitis
Sjögren's syndrome	Type 1 diabetes
Sperm & testicular autoimmunity	Ulcerative colitis (UC)
Stiff person syndrome (SPS)	Undifferentiated connective tissue disease (UCTD)
Subacute bacterial endocarditis (SBE)	Uveitis
Susac's syndrome	Vasculitis
Sympathetic ophthalmia (SO)	Vitiligo
Takayasu's arteritis	Vogt-Koyanagi-Harada Disease

One of my driving passions in life is understanding the mechanisms behind autoimmune responses, thanks in part to my own journey with an autoimmune disease. That is why, today, the bulk of my practice is auto-immune related.

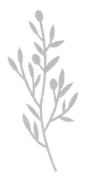

> **My patients kept getting bloodwork done and being told, "Your labs are normal."**

Most of my patients come to me after fighting the effects of chronic inflammation for decades. Sadly, they had no clue that was what they were even fighting until inflammation had done its damage, and their bodies revolted.

They kept getting bloodwork done and being told, "Your labs are normal."

But they knew better. They knew that the pain, fatigue, gut issues, skin concerns, and depression they were feeling were anything but "normal."

If you're a person who kept fighting when your doctor told you what you were feeling was just a "normal" part of aging or your inevitable cross to bear, you are amazing. This book is for you, and I'm honored to be a part of your journey.

Asking the Right Questions

There is no doubt that autoimmune diseases such as lupus, fibromyalgia, celiac disease, Hashimoto's thyroiditis, and type 1 diabetes are on the rise. Still, researchers at the CDC are stumped as to why. Experts will admit that "environmental factors are at play," but that's about as willing as they are to acknowledge that something is very, very wrong.[153]

What is making the immune system revolt against the very thing it is designed to protect? What is causing our bodies to mistake friend for foe and turn on itself?

The majority of my patients with autoimmune diseases come to me because they are tired of the generic answer: "You have XYZ disease, and you will have it for the rest of your life."

That answer is not good enough, and it certainly doesn't help explain why the soldiers that once guarded the gate are now attacking their own temple (since that's exactly what your body is).

Patients walk through my door, looking for answers. Within the first few minutes, I typically uncover more about *why* this is happening to them than they experienced in years of seeking conventional medical advice.

I'm no magician or a brilliant medical mind. I simply ask the same questions that other functional medicine professionals ask—commonsense stuff like:

- "Are you pooping?"
- "Do you know what's in your personal care products?"
- "How does your body react when you eat bread?"
- "What was your childhood like?"
- "What is your typical stress level on any given day?"
- "If not now, when did you feel the best in life?"

The list of questions goes on and on.

It's not rocket science. I ask about diet, bowel movements, sleep and exercise habits, past traumas and current stress levels, and community support systems.

The answers as to why their bodies are in revolt are almost always found within these six areas.

Disease development does not follow a predictable path, nor does progression ever look the same in two people. Our bodies are complex instruments with so many moving parts. All we can do is look at the fullest picture possible.

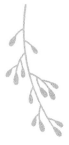

There are no drugs on the market that will "cure" your disease.

My patients have gone around the mountain for decades. They've been given pharmaceuticals after pharmaceuticals, some of which suppressed symptoms, but most never fully solved their problems.

Prescription medications have their place, and I prescribe them daily in my office, but let's get one thing straight:

There are no drugs on the market that will "cure" your disease. Perhaps except for antibiotics, many drugs are meant to be taken in perpetuity. Stop taking the medication, and whatever symptoms it was repressing all come back with a vengeance.

You may have heard stories about people who were able to successfully reverse their disease. I've witnessed it myself—patients who were able to completely stop their type 2 diabetes meds. Some people went from having painful skin conditions to seeing calm, clear skin. Some patients went from having debilitating inflammatory bowel disorders to being symptom *and* medication free. However, these miraculous stories never originated in a bottle, and they are certainly not guaranteed.

I've been faithfully following a strict diet and incorporating the lifestyle changes I recommend in this book for years, and guess what? On paper, I still have lupus. However, on most days, I am symptom-free—that is, unless a little dairy finds its way into my diet or I get run down from too much travel and not enough sleep.

I will probably have positive antibodies for lupus for the remainder of my time on Earth. That doesn't mean I can't do everything in my power not to let it affect my daily life. It's my responsibility to take steps to reduce chronic inflammation and continue to find ways to treat my body well.

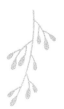

I know better, so it's my responsibility to do better.

The Lifestyle Disease Era

In the last chapter, we talked a lot about inflammation.

When chronic inflammation is never addressed, your immune system gets triggered again—and again—and again—and again. That slow-burning, festering inflammation continues to wreak havoc on your systems. The end result is never a good one.

For 20 years, my journey took the same progression as millions of others.

Every year, I felt worse.

Year after year, more things hurt, and more parts of me felt utterly broken.

Provider after provider left me deflated—and some days hopeless.

Drug after drug left me dazed and confused and not one bit better.

My voyage ultimately resulted in autoimmune disease.

Maybe you are one of the lucky ones. Perhaps your immune system has not revolted as mine did. Unfortunately, autoimmune disease isn't the only possible outcome of chronic inflammation caused by poor choices. Another route is developing a lifestyle disease.

What is a lifestyle disease? The name is pretty self-explanatory, but if you Google it, you'll find something like this:

> ### *life·style dis·ease*
> (*noun*): A medical condition or disorder regarded as being associated with how a person lives, such as heart disease, type 2 diabetes, or obesity.

That's accurate, but in my opinion, it's a little dry and doesn't quite tell the whole story. So, indulge me and allow me to define it myself:

> ### *life·style dis·ease (Dani's Definition)*
> (*noun*): A lifestyle disease is one that YOU could have prevented had you either KNOWN better or DONE better. When you know better, you must do better. If you choose to continue your bad habits, that's on you. Nobody else. Simple as that.

With so many unhealthy daily choices made by a majority of Americans, is it any surprise that the top pharmaceuticals sold in the U.S. almost exclusively target lifestyle disease symptoms? Here are the top 10 most prescribed drugs in our nation as of 2018:[154]

Drug	Most Popular	Primary Use
Lisinopril	Zestril, Prinivil	High blood pressure/anti-hypertensive
Levothyroxine	Synthroid	Hypothyroidism/low thyroid hormone
Atorvastatin (Statin)	Lipitor	Cholesterol-lowering/anti-hyperlipidemic
Metformin	Glucophage	Anti-diabetic/lower blood sugar
Simvastatin	Zocor, FloLipid	Cholesterol-lowering/anti-hyperlipidemic
Omeprazole	Prilosec	Anti-GERD/reduce heartburn
Amlodipine Besylate	Amvaz, Norvasc	High blood pressure/anti-hypertensive

Drug	Most Popular	Primary Use
Metroprolol	Lopressor, Toprol X	High blood pressure/ anti-hypertensive
Hydrocodone/ Acetaminophen	Vicodin, Lortab, Norco, Lorcet	Opioid/Analgesic
Albuterol	Proventil, Ventolin	Bronchodilator

Let's break down this list.

Three of the most popular drugs listed are for high blood pressure. This is undoubtedly a concern since it is a precursor for some terrifying lifestyle-related conditions, including cardiovascular disease and stroke, which are number one and number five in the leading causes of death in America, respectively.

The two cholesterol-lowering drugs are no surprise, since high cholesterol is positively correlated to obesity, and this nation is getting fatter and fatter. High cholesterol is also tied to the number one killer, heart disease.

Of course, there's a drug for diabetes on there—and it's not type 1 diabetes (the one that is genuinely genetic), but for type 2 diabetes only. Diabetes comes in at number seven on the top killers in America list, and it's certainly not due to type 1. Of the 10.5 percent of the population with diabetes (34.2 million people), only 1.4 million people have type 1.

Heartburn made the list because people can't be bothered to eat less or avoid foods that knowingly cause them indigestion. Or providers can't be bothered to educate their patients on the fact that the McDonald's drive-through and Big Gulp sodas are creating heartburn and disease in their bodies.

Here's an interesting fact: Do you know 20 percent of all meals are now consumed in the car? How many times have you fed your children in the car on the way to school, soccer practice, etc.?

An opioid is also in the top ten list, which is not surprising given the opioid crisis that is currently gripping our nation and destroying people's lives. People are taking pills to numb to their physical pain, but perhaps even more frequent but less talked about, their emotional pain.

People are hurting and crying out for help, and the only way they know to get by is to take a pill to numb them from feeling anything. Opioids are highly addictive. Long-term use of painkillers is also associated with a heightened risk of developing major depression. Patients using painkillers for over six months had more than a 50 percent greater chance of developing a depressive episode.

Asking for Help is the Bravest Thing You Can Do

I am passionate about suicide prevention. I have a strong family history of suicide and lived through experiencing depression myself. I am now on the board of the American Foundation for Suicide Prevention and do my best to get the word out that help is available and that struggling alone doesn't have to be your reality.

If you or someone you know is in crisis, I implore you to reach out. You can call the suicide crisis prevention hotline at **800-273-8255, text TALK to 741-741, and visit their website at AFSP.org** for resources, information, and encouragement. You are not alone, and there are people who care and want to help!

The even greater issue hidden within is that suicide is currently the tenth leading cause of death in this country. Even more terrifying and heartbreaking, suicide is the second leading cause of death for young people between ages 10 and 24.

Now, let's look at this in comparison to something you hear about more frequently. You can't go into a CVS, Wal-Mart, or Target without seeing marketing for free flu shots and bribes with gift cards and more. Half of the articles during cold and flu season (and now COVID-19) every year are fearmongering "end of the world as we know it" level reporting.

The flu is nothing to sneeze at, but consider this: In 2017, the number of confirmed influenza related deaths in Americans ages 10 to 24 was **241** people. Compare that to the **6,769** young people ages 10 to 24 who deliberately took their own life in that same year.

Another drug on the list is used to treat hypothyroidism, which occurs when the thyroid doesn't make enough of the hormone called thyroxine (T4). The most common cause of hypothyroidism is an autoimmune disease known as Hashimoto's thyroiditis. According to the Mayo Clinic, "doctors don't know what causes your immune system to attack your thyroid gland."

For those with Hashimoto's, that's certainly not very comforting, is it?

Unfortunately, it gets worse. MedicineNet, a popular website in operation since 1995 that provides "doctor-produced health and medical information," actually has this statement on their website: "Since Hashimoto's thyroiditis is an autoimmune disorder, it cannot be prevented."

I call BS on this.

If you weren't born with it, you *can* prevent it!

If you weren't born with it, you *can* prevent it!

Allopathic (modern) medicine promotes the idea that autoimmune disease is *inevitable*! And *this* is the limiting mindset with which the medical profession approaches treating our bodies and our lives.

Type 2 diabetes is now considered an autoimmune disease. Eczema is classified as autoimmune. Can such conditions be prevented in all cases? No. But I'll tell you this. **I've had patients be completely healed from their ailments. No medications, no flare-ups. Total remission.**

Don't ever let *anyone* tell you that you cannot be healed or that because your parents were sick, you will be, too.

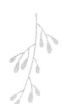

Don't let limiting beliefs stop you from living a better and more joy-filled life.

Don't let limiting beliefs stop you from living a better and more joy-filled life.

Don't let lies rob you of the mindset it takes to be Wild & Well.

Nelson Mandela once said, "It always seems impossible until it's done." I'll add a quote by Helen Keller to this:

"Optimism is the faith that leads to achievement. Nothing can be done without hope and confidence."

Do you believe that you can be well? Do you *want* to be well?

My patients want to be well, but before they found functional medicine, no one was offering them a way out.

I had a four-year-old come me with a juvenile arthritis diagnosis handed down to her at age two. The source was unknown, and her doctors were unwilling to get to the bottom of the diagnosis. Instead, they told the parents of a toddler that her body would struggle with this disease and the stiffness she was experiencing for the rest of her life, and they aren't sure why. Then they put her on Methotrexate, Embrel, and Humira over the next year, with no plan to find the root cause that would explain why a two-year-old would have a lifetime diagnosis like juvenile arthritis.

As I sat and listened to her parents' heartbreak and struggle to come to terms with the diagnosis, my heart broke for them.

If you are struggling with a diagnosis and your doctors have given you the equivalent of a shrug and "we will see you in six months," then you need to do three things right away.

1. Find a new doctor (don't forget WE work for YOU as healthcare providers).

2. Find hope for the future.

3. Find and implement an action plan (because hope is great but also useless without a strategy).

You are *not* defined by your diagnosis, and your future is *not* pre-determined.

If you are alive today, there is a way out. But that way is not *around* the problem with Band-Aid solutions. The way out is working *through* the problem by finding and eliminating root causes.

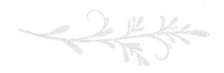

The Toxic Straw That Broke the Camel's Back

We are headed into Part Two, but before we dive into which lifestyle decisions heal and which ones harm, let me ask a few simple questions:

Are you going to die young *just* because you eat dairy and gluten?

Are you doing to develop heart disease because you didn't exercise enough?

Are you going to develop cancer entirely because you use Bluetooth headphones or have anxiety?

Let's not be dramatic.

There is not one single lifestyle habit that is "killing" you all on its own. Life is stressful for everyone, and no one is perfect. No matter how hard you try to make good choices, there will be times when you: eat things you shouldn't, think negative thoughts, feel stressed, fail to get enough sleep, get constipated, don't drink enough water, get a second helping of dessert, shower with unfiltered water, and much more.

The problem isn't each one of those decisions—the problem is *all* of them combined.

Take a person who eats the SAD diet, and then tack on poor sleep habits, sedentary lifestyle, chronic constipation, elevated stress levels, adverse childhood experiences, and toxic relationships. Eventually, one additional poor lifestyle choice could be the proverbial last straw.

Your body is amazing, but it can only do so much.

Every decision you make matters.

Every. Single. One.

Are you ready to make better choices—one habit and one step at a time?

If so, I believe you are ready to begin Part Two, which will break down the six lifestyle areas that have the most dramatic effects on your health and the health of your family.

I want you to live a genuinely Wild & Well life. I want you to feel excited to jump out of bed in the morning.

I'm not here to tell you to "find a job you love, and you'll never work a day in your life."

I'm also not here to tell you that "if it tastes good, spit it out."

I am a realist, and I will be the first to admit that I fail every single day. I say things I shouldn't, I have a sweet tooth, and I all too often allow work and personal issues to stress me out.

I'm not asking you or expecting you to be perfect. I'm asking you to go into Part Two with an open mind and an open heart and be honest with yourself. In Part Two, you will need to answer some tough questions, but the good news is there is no graded test at the end. I won't call you up and ask you to recite all of the main points or expect you to never eat another slice of pizza or cake ever again.

I'm human, and I'm pretty sure you are, too.

So, human to human, I know you are strong, and I know you want to feel better. And if you'll let me, I'd like to help you get closer to that goal.

wild & well Rx

Dani Williamson, MSN, FNP

℞ Patient Name: ....

Age: ....   Date: ....

1. Most of us were *not* born sick, so we should not live our lives content to be sick.

2. Realize that what you turn on you can turn back off... I am living proof of that.

3. Make the decision to live the life God gave you to enjoy. If you are alive today, then you can be on the road to recovery.

4. Decide to believe that you are worthy, no matter how hard the journey may be. Mindset is 90 percent of health.

5. Feel hope, even if you have an autoimmune disorder. No matter where you are now, you can begin to decrease inflammation with the steps in Part Two.

6. Settle on a strategy to begin to heal your body. One day at a time. And no, hope is not a strategy.

7. Remind yourself that there is no single thing that causes a chronic lifestyle disease. It's years of toxic buildup.

8. Get help. If you don't have family support, join our Facebook community (Inside Out Healing From Within), ask friends, and decide that you are worthy of being healthy and whole.

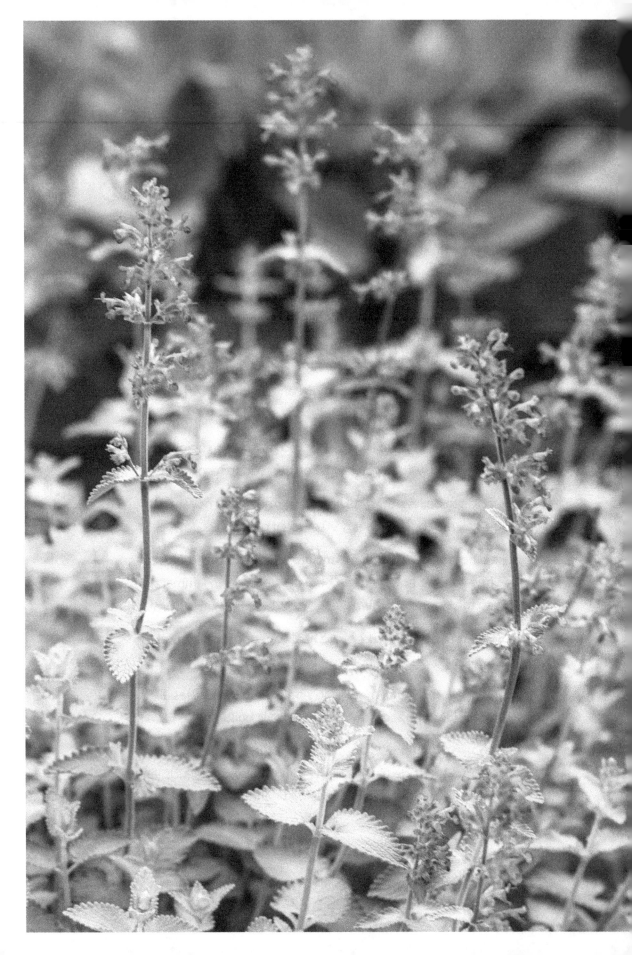

PART TWO

commonsense
action

Attention!

If you only read one chapter of this book, it needs to be this one.

This chapter is the key to unlocking your healthiest you.

Had just one person asked me 24 years sooner, "What are you eating?" my story would have been so much different and far less painful.

CHAPTER 5

eat well

"The whiter your bread, the sooner you're dead."
GRANDMA MILDRED

Our health is a mess. People are in more pain and struggle at earlier ages than ever before. How did it come to this? What is the root cause of the rising rates of chronic and autoimmune diseases? There are multiple contributing factors that we have already discussed and will continue to examine. However, the primary reason is not hard to determine.

It's because of food.

What goes down your pie hole will either heal or kill you. That may not be tactful, but the truth rarely is.

The majority of food at the grocery store and your favorite restaurants and drive-throughs is no longer food. It may *look* like real food, but it is processed, inflammatory, and mostly devoid of nutrition. As much as 70 percent of what we eat is denatured and nutritionally empty.

Since we are what we eat, that's a problem.

What even happens to food during processing? The scary thing is we don't know for sure. Despite the global mass consumption of processed foods, we still aren't sure of the extent of chemical modifications that nutrients undergo during processing and how those alterations affect body chemistry.[155]

When food manufacturers *do* discover a chemical or biochemical reaction that adversely alters food quality or safety, their response is to add *more*—more acidulants (chemical compounds designed to emulate the taste of real food and make it more shelf stable), more chelating agents (additives that increase shelf life), more preservatives, and more artificial flavors.[156]

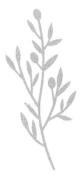

It is estimated that the average American takes in about 2,000 pounds of food a year!

Have you ever wondered why your food from a famous chicken fast food restaurant, or your biscuits and gravy from another famous nation-wide chain taste the same in Franklin, TN as they do in Sacramento, CA? It's because of those additives listed above. Your food is a chemistry experiment, a science project.

Is it any wonder, then, why a person's life span is determined by the combined effects of both genetics *and* environmental factors such as diet?[157] Studies suggest that genetics accounts for just 20 to 30 percent of an individual's chance of reaching age 85.[158] Decades-old research indicates that diet accounts for about 30 percent of the risk of developing diseases such as cancer.[159] Dietary choices are also considered to be primary risk factors in the development of cardiovascular disease—the number one killer for both men and women.[160]

We Americans tend to look to other cultures when it comes to discovering the "secret" to living longer, healthier lives that are free from disease. Monaco is the country at the top of the life expectancy list, with an average of 89.52 years. The island of Okinawa in Japan also is often cited as having the stellar life expectancy rates. It is referred to as a "blue zone," an area where residents live longer than most other people in the world.[161]

Coming in at an unimpressive number 43 out of 195 on the list of life expectancy by country, the U.S. seems to be falling behind. Our nation's current life expectancy is age 76 for men and age 81 for women. However, there is a group of people living right here in America who seem to have figured out some things that the rest of the country has not.

The picturesque, small town of Loma Linda in California has one of the highest life expectancies in the world. If you are a resident, you are ten times more likely to live to 100 than the rest of us. The average life expectancy of men is 89, and women live to age 91 on average.

That is ten years more than the national average!

Is it the balmy California weather? The prevalence of backyard swimming pools? It is far more likely that the reason is that Loma Linda is home to a thriving population

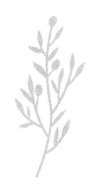

Genetics is only a small part of the story. Your environment and lifestyle choices are critical to your life's outcome!

of Seventh-day Adventists. This religious group places great importance on treating the body like a temple. Adventists do not drink alcohol, smoke, or eat meat, and they get plenty of exercise. They are a tight-knit community that treats each other like family. They also prioritize the Sabbath as a day to de-stress and find peace.[162]

In other words, they eat well, move well, de-stress well, and commune well—and I'm taking liberties here, but I bet they also poop and sleep well.

Skeptics and opponents of unprocessed, unmodified foods (such as food manufacturers, fast food chains, and companies like Monsanto) love to point out that if you remove murders and fatal car crashes, the U.S. would have one of the best life expectancy rates in the world.

According to them, we are just fine!

Or maybe our healthcare is to blame. After all, America is falling behind because of the lack of universal healthcare, right?

Interestingly, in 2016, after millions received coverage under Obamacare, American life expectancy went down for the first time in over 20 years. I'm not suggesting that Obamacare was responsible for anyone's demise. What I am saying is that, logically speaking, life expectancy numbers can be skewed by many things.

> **Chemical-laden foods, synthetic ingredients, rancid processed meats and fats, and genetically produced crops are linked to inflammation. Inflammation is connected to every major disease. Who prefers to live a life of any length that is full of pain and illness?**

In actuality, it doesn't matter whether our country ranks at the top or the bottom of any list—because here is the *real* truth:

Chemical-laden foods, synthetic ingredients, rancid processed meats and fats, and genetically produced crops are linked to inflammation. Inflammation is connected to every major disease. Who prefers to live a life of *any* length that is full of pain and illness?

This is not rocket science.

Nothing "just happens" out of the blue when it concerns your health. There is a tipping point, and that tipping point is different for everyone. A poor diet full of fake, processed, packaged, bagged, canned, man-made food is where it begins for most.

People who are skeptical of eating healthy or simply don't want to change old habits love to bring up their 98-year-old grandma who "smoked until the day she died and drank six sodas a day."

Good for Grandma! She got lucky.

I'm not interested in relying on luck as a long-term health strategy. Those of us who don't want to gamble with the one life we have on this earth must undergo a conscious awakening and experience an about-face to find the path back to health.

To help you become fully awake, let's retrace our steps and find out when the food supply became so toxic and inflammatory.

A Brief History of Food

People have been preserving foods for millennia. However, the industrialization of food has taken food-keeping techniques and mass production to the extreme. They are so pervasive that they have virtually destroyed farming, one of the noblest trades since the beginning of time.

The farming of today looks nothing like it did not so long ago. Large corporations have taken over the cultivation of our land, and they have put processes in place that allow them to sell nutritionally empty, fake food to us at a staggering profit for them.[163]

The growing demand for fast food and convenience store snacks only makes the problem worse, because the more we buy, the more crap they make. Processed food satisfies our cravings, it's cheap, and it's convenient, but we are paying a high price for these meager benefits.

You name the disease, and I will wager that food is a significant factor in its development—autoimmune disease, metabolic disease, obesity, cancer, heart disease, mental health conditions, and more. Not to mention antibiotic resistance and the stripping of healthy gut bacteria.

They Do WHAT to My Food?

While food manufacturers claim that decontaminating foods via *irradiation* is safe, the chemical composition and nutritional content of food can change after exposure to ionizing radiation. Chemical by-products are often formed in irradiated food and very few of them have been adequately studied for toxicity. Critics say that all the process does is mask but not remedy unsanitary conditions at plants that led to the need for the procedure in the first place.

Prior to the 20th century, all food was "organic" because crops were grown without the use of chemical ripening or fertilizers, food irradiation, food additives, or genetically modified ingredients.[164]

In sharp contrast, we must now rely on multiple labels on even our fresh produce to ensure that the food isn't made with dangerous chemicals in unsafe conditions.

We must now rely on multiple labels on even our fresh produce to ensure that the food isn't made with dangerous chemicals in unsafe conditions.

The idea of a grocery store would be a mind-blowing concept for anyone living in the thousands of years before the first self-service grocery store opened in 1916—which was a Piggly Wiggly in Memphis, Tennessee. For the vast majority of history, the inhabitants of cities and villages relied upon the farmers and herders who hocked their crops, dry goods, and animal products at local markets and in town squares.

At the turn of the 19th century in America, things mostly resembled that old way of life, and 95 percent of families still lived in rural areas. However, by 1900, that dropped to 40 percent, with the majority moving to the growing cities.

The shift to the city brought with it a complete transformation of the food system. Food producers began using industrialized methods of mass production. Synthetic pesticides were also developed, and the use of chemicals in farming expanded greatly in the late 1800s.[165]

As the population grew in our country, so did technological advances. The household refrigerator was invented in 1913 by Fred Wolf, and on the surface, what a great invention it was. However, a 2005 study out of Penn State University found that it takes only eight days in the refrigerator for fresh spinach to lose 47 percent of its folate and other nutrients.[166] So, food may not spoil as quickly, but it's certainly not going to pack the nutritional punch it should.

Truth Bomb

Fresh produce, such as spinach, loses almost half of its nutrients after a week in the fridge.

The population shift, combined with the rise of industry, changed agricultural methods forever. The Great Depression was arguably the biggest deathblow to the "old ways" of doing life in America. Farms went under, and when the American economy reemerged, large corporations owned much of the farmland once owned by families.

The World Wars did their part to transform eating as well. After the wars, food makers needed a place to sell the foods they had been making for soldiers (such as Spam, dehydrated potatoes, instant coffee, and powdered fruit juices). They targeted the American housewife, marketing fake food as "packaged food cuisine."

Women went to work outside the homes en masse for the first time, and TV dinners were on the rise as "latchkey kids" became the norm, not the exception. I was one of those latchkey kids who was mesmerized by aluminum-tray TV dinners (my favorite part was that lump of tan food they called dessert). Frozen pot pies and frozen pizzas were also staples in my home.

And so mass-produced, processed food became widely accepted and even beloved—and with its rise came the need for faster, cheaper methods of growing, harvesting, and preserving ingredients from the earth.

We started making Frankenfoods and stuffing them with the cheapest fillers possible that would still allow them to be labeled as edible.

We started making Frankenfoods and stuffing them with the cheapest fillers possible that would still allow them to be labeled as edible.

For example, today's top four global crops are corn, soy, rice, and wheat. When foods aren't eaten in their fresh, whole, one-ingredient forms, you can expect them to be made with one or more of these four foods. If you pick up a package in the middle aisles of your supermarket, it would be shocking not to see one or all of these plant-based derivatives in the ingredients.

Do you think people in the 1800s daily ate foods containing hidden soy?

When the American Indians were teaching European settlers how to fertilize sandy soil to grow corn, could they have imagined that, one day, corn would be used to make an artificial sweetener that has helped lead to this country's diabetes and obesity epidemics?[167]

The Plant-Based Trap

Seeing the phrase "plant-based" on a package doesn't mean it's healthy. High-fructose corn syrup is plant-based. Frosted Flakes are plant-based. Fast-food French fries are plant-based. Don't let a trend fool you into eating inflammatory foods!

The madness must stop. It's time to take back control of our health—and that requires us to know the truth so we can choose better. Industrialization and modern farming practices are to blame for America's health crisis, not genetics or bad luck.

The Seven Most Inflammatory Foods

Chronic inflammation is responsible for most of my patients' pain and discomfort. I suffered the debilitating effects of inflammation for years with no clue that food was the source of my agony. For many others, however, the symptoms are not so obvious. Chronic inflammation is so insidious that you may not even know you are suffering from it until it manifests in the form of an auto-immune disease, cancer, or other devastating condition.

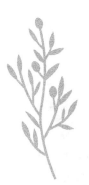

> **One of the greatest lies we've been led to believe is that as we age, we are supposed to hurt.**

Or, you may have symptoms that you simply consider to be "normal." You might have gotten used to feeling tired and achy. You are accustomed to the daily bloating and gas, and you consider your insomnia and mood swings to be inevitable. Here's a news flash for you: Your body was *not* designed to feel those things.

One of the greatest lies we've been led to believe is that as we age, we are supposed to hurt. Or we could say: One of the greatest lies we have been led to believe is that joint pain is a 'normal' part of aging.

We were designed for a wildly vibrant, full life with a body that functions as the good Lord intended. But it's up to you to make better choices, remove the poisons that are destroying your health, and start taking in healing fuel.

If you want to feel well, the first and most critical step is to eat well.

We'll cover what foods are best, but the real key is to identify what *not* to eat. One of the first things I do with new patients is a full food sensitivity panel that gives them a complete list of foods to avoid due to their unique sensitivities.

I've never seen two identical panels, but seven foods are known to cause more problems and inflammation than others. Therefore, I have my patients eliminate these foods right away, long before their results are back from the lab. Even if you do not do food sensitivity testing, eliminating these top seven foods is critical to beginning your healing journey, in my opinion.

These foods are proven to create an inflammatory and/or immune response in our bodies and fan the flames for slow-burning systemic inflammation. Not everyone has a food allergy or sensitivity to all of them. Still, every one of these foods has the potential to create inflammation, gut dysfunction, and more.

I call them the Sinister Seven.

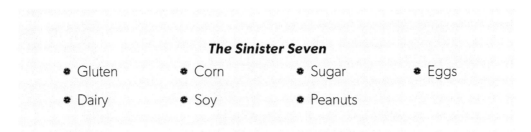

The Sinister Seven

- Gluten
- Corn
- Sugar
- Eggs
- Dairy
- Soy
- Peanuts

It has been common knowledge in the functional medicine world for years that certain foods create inflammation and contribute to widespread chronic health issues. This is not groundbreaking knowledge never revealed until now. In fact, I have been recommending JJ Virgin's book, *The Virgin Diet*, to my patients for years. She also advises the removal of these seven foods from any diet.

Like JJ, I quickly noticed that most of my patients were reacting to the

Sinister Seven. When JJ released her book, it was a game-changer for me. I started recommending it to every single patient who walked through my doors. Personally, gluten, dairy, and eggs have been on my food sensitivity results for almost a decade. Even after removing them, I still react to them when tested.

These are not newly created foods invented by food manufacturers. They have been eaten in abundance for as long as people have been eating. So, why are they a problem now?

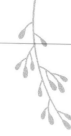

Food used to be one ingredient. Salmon. Rice. Apple. Spinach. Almonds.

That is a complicated answer. Part of the problem is what's included in these foods and how processed they've become.

Food used to be one ingredient. Salmon. Rice. Apple. Spinach. Almonds.

Now it takes a degree in chemistry to pronounce all of the crap in our foods.

Let's say you go to Burger King and decide to skip the burger and opt for their BK Broiler Chicken Sandwich. It's flame-broiled, so you assume it's better. Here's a list of the ingredients in the chicken alone:

> BK BROILER® CHICKEN BREAST PATTY: Boneless chicken breast with rib meat, water, seasoning (salt, chicken stock, flavoring, maltodextrin, and autolyzed yeast), partially hydrogenated **soybean oil** and sodium phosphates. Glazed with water, seasoning (maltodextrin, salt, chicken stock, hydrolyzed **soy protein**, flavors, modified food starch, methylcellulose gum, monosodium glutamate, **soy sauce** (**wheat, soybeans,** salt) chicken fat, hydrolyzed **wheat gluten**, xanthan gum, natural smoke flavor, partially hydrogenated **soybean oil**, **butter** (**cream**, salt) **hydrolyzed corn gluten**, autolyzed yeast extract, **buttermilk**, **corn syrup solids**, thiamine hydrochloride, citric acid, lactic acid, caramel color, disodium inosinate disodium guanylate vegetable stock (carrot, onion, celery, paprika, and tocopherol) and partially hydrogenated **soybean oil**.

Pretty gross. If the ingredients of your broiled chicken include more than chicken, herbs, and spices, you are forcing your body to fight a battle against dysfunction and disease that it will ultimately lose.

The rest of this chapter is devoted to the top seven inflammatory foods and why they may be causing you to live less than your best life. I'm not saying you have to give them all up immediately and never eat them again. What I am saying is there's a strong chance that several (or all) of these foods are causing your body to suffer.

If you are asking yourself, "But do I really have to change what I eat?" let me go ahead and burst your bubble. *Yes, you do.* Lots of mainstream, fad diets prey on people's food addictions by claiming, "You don't have to give up your favorite foods!"

That may be true if your goal is temporary weight loss. However, if your goal is health, disease reversal, pain-free days, and a Wild & Well life, then it's time for some real talk.

Pro Tip: To help reframe your mind and gain a new perspective, instead of asking, "What favorite foods do I have to give up?" think, "What healthy foods can become my new favorites?"

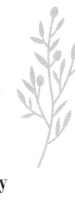

The foods you choose will heal you or kill you—and it really is your choice. It's all about perspective. So, let's get started.

1. Gluten, the Gut Grenade

We are going to spend more time on gluten than the other seven. The reason is because of bread. Ah, bread—the soft, sumptuous, fluffy, beige delight whose mere smell can cause us to salivate without warning.

We start shoving bread and gluten-containing products into our mouths just about as soon as we can chew, and for most of us, the love affair never ends. Unfortunately, it's a toxic, one-sided relationship. So, consider this your intervention. And before you ask, your body is not the problem.

"Give us this day our daily bread."

It's not you, it's gluten.

I often hear, "But Jesus ate bread!" In Matthew 6:11, Jesus even mentions bread in the famous Sermon on the Mount as part of the Lord's Prayer:

"Give us this day our daily bread… "

Yep, that's right—bread is not inherently evil! Civilizations have been munching on loaves for as long as history has been recorded. Jesus broke bread with his disciples and followers, but his bread was made from one of only three possible strains, one of which was called einkorn.

Einkorn's recorded use goes all the way back to the Paleolithic era, where hunter-gatherers in the Far East harvested it from the wild. In 10,000 B.C., the first farmers planted einkorn, and it began to grow domestically. Compared to modern wheat, ancient wheats, such as einkorn, are better in every way. Here are just a few of the best things about einkorn wheat:

- It's the only wheat strain never hybridized (cross-bred to create new strains).

- Some people who are sensitive to modern strains of wheat show little to no reaction to Einkorn wheat in small amounts.

- It contains 40 percent more protein, 15 percent less starch, and 20 percent more fiber than modern wheat.

- Einkorn has twice the antioxidant (cancer-fighting) activity as modern wheat.

- Finally, it contains 42 percent more zinc, 80 percent more manganese, and 25 percent more magnesium than newer wheat strains.

Wheat has evolved from three strains to over 25,000 species today, most of which were created labs to be disease resistant or produce higher

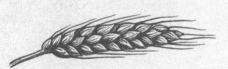

ANCIENT WHEAT:
naturally smaller grains

MODERN WHEAT: fatter, genetically modified grains

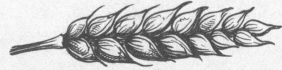

yields. While those are admirable goals, breeding wheat to create new strains (a process called *wheat hybridization*) may have led to the rapidly growing prevalence of gluten intolerance and celiac disease.

Bread, flour, baked goods. Even if you buy organic, it's all hybridized.

Before hybridization became commonplace, wheat was five to six feet tall (think flowing, amber waves of grain), and the head on the wheat was very small. In an effort to produce bigger yields to feed more people, they started creating higher-yield wheat that didn't have to grow as tall so they could harvest its big head sooner. The end result is called "dwarf wheat" due to its diminutive size compared to the ancient strains.

> **Did you know a piece of whole wheat toast increases your blood sugar more than a can of soda or a candy bar?**

Being able to feed more people sounds like a great idea! The problem was they didn't check to see if this new hybridized, fat-headed, stubby wheat was still edible.

It turns out it really isn't. The gluten contained in modern wheat is essentially indigestible—hence the meteoric rise of gut-related conditions such as IBS and Crohn's, not to mention chronic inflammation and autoimmune disease.

Modern wheat also contains a "super carbohydrate" called amylopectin A that is shown to be one of the greatest contributors to the insulin resistance and type 2 diabetes epidemic in this country. After just eight weeks of eating amylopectin-rich starches, the insulin response was 100 percent greater in mice when compared to mice that were fed amylose, another starch found in whole plant-based foods.[168]

A study conducted on human participants had similar results. Researchers at the Beltsville Human Nutrition Research Center found that men who consumed a diet containing 34 percent of their calories from amylose had significantly lower glucose and insulin responses compared with those consuming the same number of calories from the super carb amylopectin.[169]

Refined grains tend to be digested more quickly, leading to blood sugar spikes. These surges are followed by drops, which increase cravings and create a vicious, harmful cycle of food addiction that leads to the development of type 2 diabetes.[170]

But aren't complex carbs like whole wheat supposed to be good for you?

Well, here's the deal. According to findings presented by Dr. William Davis in his groundbreaking book, *Wheat Belly*, about 75 percent of the complex carbohydrate in wheat is amylopectin and just 25 percent is amylose. Here is how Dr. Davis explains the digestion of a piece of reportedly "healthy" whole wheat bread:

> "Amylopectin is efficiently digested by amylase to glucose, while amylose is much less efficiently digested, some of it making its way to the colon undigested. Thus, the complex carbohydrate amylopectin is rapidly converted to glucose and absorbed into the bloodstream and, because it is most efficiently digested, is mainly responsible for wheat's blood-sugar-increasing effects."

To add to the serious health risks, modern wheat is also soaked in Monsanto's industry-dominating herbicide called Roundup (glyphosate) just days before it is harvested. This practice is called *desiccating*, and it began in Scotland in the 1980s. Scottish farmers had trouble getting their grains to dry evenly, so they came up with a plan to evenly kill the crop (with glyphosate) a week or so before the harvest so the grain would be uniformly dried and ready for processing.

That sounds like an efficient idea. Sadly, it also sounds like farmers now spray our food with certified-cancer-causing poison right before they serve it to us. And that's not conspiracy theory talk or fringe science. In 2015, the World Health Organization's (WHO) International Agency for Research on Cancer (IARC) formally released findings indicating that glyphosate is a "probable human carcinogen."[171]

But don't farmers know better? No, they don't, thanks to companies like Monsanto that spend countless dollars to promote their fabricated studies that prove how "safe" and "biodegradable" their poison is. When it comes to sourcing conventional grains, millers will tell you that it's almost impossible to find grains that have not been sprayed with glyphosate just before harvesting. Much of the industry seems to operate according to a "don't ask, don't tell" policy when it comes to desiccating. (It's worth noting that, as mentioned above, this practice applies to crops grown in other countries as well. Sadly, it's a common misconception that food grown outside the U.S. is chemical-free.)

Bromine is now in our bread as well. Bromine is a toxic chemical element classified as a halogen, the same group containing poisons such as chlorine and fluoride. Bromated flour makes the dough elastic, enabling it to stand up to bread hoods better.

Sounds okay—until you realize that bromine mimics iodine.

> **Bromine messes with our iodine levels and leads to thyroid issues.**

In a nutshell, what that means is bromine blocks your glandular receptor sites and interferes with the metabolism of iodine, which then leads to a host of issues, including thyroid disorders. **My patients rarely have normal iodine levels.** Most of them need an iodine supplement to increase their levels.

Bromine is just bad news. In animal studies, scientists have even shown that bromine negatively impacts the amount of iodine transferred to a mother's young via breast milk.[172]

Surprisingly, wheat is not yet widely genetically modified. Monsanto was set to release a glyphosate-resistant genetically engineered strain (Roundup Ready™ Wheat) back in 2004 but soon after withdrew their EPA application.[173] But that will eventually change. Environmental risk assessments conducted by Monsanto have "proven" that, nutritionally speaking, genetically modified (GM) wheat is comparable to modern wheat. *Gee, how comforting.* GM wheat has also been approved for use in food and animal feed. So now, it's just a matter of time.

Are you mad yet? You should be! I was furious when I first discovered these practices. We're feeding this crap to our loved ones, to our children—but the truth will not remain hidden.

We've talked about wheat, but now let's take a deeper dive into the world of gluten.

MUCKING UP YOUR INSIDES

We all know someone who suffers from gluten issues. Gluten such a common buzzword now that it's impossible to escape it. I know the word means a lot to me, since gluten is one of the main reasons why I suffered endlessly for over two decades.

This may be hard to believe—considering its pervasiveness in our society—but the term "gluten-free diet" did not appear in U.S. pop culture until 2005. Since then, it has surpassed both the low-carb and low-fat diets in terms of search frequency and popularity.

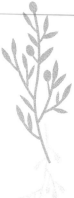

There are 3 million Americans with celiac disease and as many as 20 million more who may be suffering from non-celiac gluten sensitivity.

The market for gluten-free foods and beverages is colossal and growing at exponential rates. According to consumer goods market research company Packaged Facts, it's currently a $4.2 billion market and only getting bigger.

Why all the fuss over gluten?

The leader in gluten research is Dr. Alessio Fasano, a pediatric gastroenterologist and the director of the Center for Celiac Research who wrote the phenomenal book, *Gluten Freedom*. He says that there is only a fraction of people who can eat gluten without suffering any acute symptoms. They don't experience any bloating, joint pain, or fatigue. They don't feel sluggish or feel as though they just swallowed a lead balloon. They aren't hit with the sudden urge for a mid-morning or afternoon nap. I am definitely *not* one of those people.

They're the lucky ones—and their "luck" may have a lot to do with the health and integrity of their guts.[174]

Another even smaller fraction of the U.S. population has been diagnosed with celiac disease. It is reported that one in 133 people have celiac, which is an autoimmune disease that damages the villi of the small intestine and interferes with absorption of nutrients from food, causing serious health problems if undiagnosed. The actual number of diagnosed cases of celiac is rare, but it's on the rise. That should concern us.

What's even more concerning is that another sizable portion of the population has no business eating gluten—but they still do. According to Dr. Fasano, these are the approximately 6 to 7 percent of Americans who suffer from something called non-celiac gluten sensitivity. Others estimate the number to be closer to 13 percent, but it's a hard number to nail down. Since there is no biomarker for diagnosing the condition, the only way to diagnose it is to show or determine that a patient has a *definite* reaction to gluten but does *not* have celiac disease or a wheat allergy.

Non-celiac gluten sensitivity (or just gluten sensitivity) is referred to as a reaction to ingesting gluten-containing grains. The symptoms of gluten sensitivity can include almost everything: from gut issues such as diarrhea, bloating, cramping, and abdominal pain to skin issues such as eczema and rashes to behavioral issues such as ADD, ADHD, anxiety, and brain fog. Other symptoms include anemia, joint pain, osteoporosis, and leg numbness.[175]

Recent research shows that gluten sensitivity is a different clinical entity totally from celiac disease. It doesn't result in the intestinal inflammation that leads to the flattening of the microvilli.[176]

So, it's not going to kill you—at least not quickly. Instead:

Eating gluten when you have non-celiac gluten sensitivity will lead to the slow-burning, chronic inflammation that will eventually lead to the disease that could kill you.

Gluten, the complex and ancient protein and the main component of wheat, developed alongside humans throughout many thousands of years. A very strange and unique protein, gluten is naturally found in barley, wheat, and rye. Gluten and its close relatives secalin and hordein are the only proteins that we cannot fully digest.

With up to 334,000 genes, wheat provides us with an extremely complicated genetic maze to untangle. That's a lot of genome to consider. Wheat is more complicated than we are, since humans have just 20,000 to 25,000 genes.

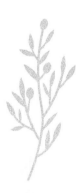

Eating gluten when you have non-celiac gluten sensitivity will lead to the slow-burning, chronic inflammation that will eventually lead to the disease that could kill you.

The history of humans and the evolution of celiac disease and gluten sensitivity are intertwined. Humans stayed in one place 10,000 years ago to plant and harvest crops and gather animals into domestic herds, and then the slow growth of agriculture led to larger societies. That's around the time when wild strains such as einkorn wheat began to be grown domestically. Since then, the genetic profile of wheat has only gotten more complicated.

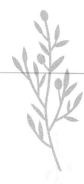

Gluten makes foods fatter, fluffier and softer, which is ironic since that's exactly what eating wheat bread does to humans!

Gluten proteins have little nutritional value, but, thanks to their unique viscoelasticity, they play a pivotal role in the production of bread and baked goods. In fact, bread companies put *additional* gluten in bread to make it rise faster and higher, so humans are consuming far more gluten than our ancestors, even if we eat the same amount of bread.

Gluten helps foods maintain their shape, acting as a glue that holds food together. When you mix water with glutenous flour, the gluten proteins form a sticky network that create a glue-like consistency that makes the dough elastic and gives bread the ability to rise when baked.

In fact, gluten literally means "glue" in Latin, which is fitting considering what it does to your intestinal tract.

If you look at gluten under a microscope, you may be much less apt to eat it. It's one giant, gluey mess and therefore no wonder why our bodies start to feel weighed down and stuck and slow.

As Hippocrates said, all disease begins in the gut. When you eat gluten, your gut has to cut through all of that glue, and remember that your digestive enzymes can't even fully digest gluten. So where does it all end up?

Stuck inside you.

Things get a little more complicated when you factor in the fact that gluten is addictive.[177] If you go to Cracker Barrel (and, oh, how I *love* Cracker Barrel), it's easy to eat three or four biscuits without batting an eye. Glutenous bread releases opioid-like compounds and therefore acts like a morphine derivative in your body, which means that the more you eat, the more you want.[178] Your blood sugar spikes, you feel that sugar high, but then comes the crash—and suddenly you want more, more, more.

On the flip side of the coin, going "gluten free" is not some health or weight loss panacea. I have patients who go gluten free and gain ten pounds. They come into my office dejected and moan, "But Dani, I thought I was supposed to *lose* weight, not gain it!"

Going gluten free is not as simple as it sounds, because remember the multi-billion-dollar, gluten-free food market? You know how they are making their billions? By marketing gluten-free junk. Waffles, cookies, and cakes are not suddenly good for you just because they don't contain gluten.

"Gluten Free" Doesn't Mean "Healthy"

Going gluten free is not a quick fix or a health panacea. Ice cream is gluten free. Cheetos are gluten free. Skittles are gluten free. Candy corn is gluten free. Fruity Pebbles and Lucky Charms are gluten free.

Another issue is the label "gluten free" is used very liberally. The FDA defines the term and regulates over its use when it comes to food manufacturers. However, when it comes to restaurants using the term, you have to take their word for it. A restaurant may make their "gluten free" pizza dough on the exact same surface they just made the wheat-based one. Even worse, they may be dishonest, and the only way you'll find out is the telltale GI distress you feel from a few hours to a few days after a glutenous meal.

THE RISE OF CELIAC

People with celiac disease produce antibodies that, in combination with hormone-like substances called cytokines and the direct effect of immune cells, attack the intestines and flatten the villi, leading to malabsorption and illness. It's as serious as it sounds, but celiac disease is still fairly rare (currently affects about 1 percent of the U.S. population).

However, it's on the rise. The reason is because, according to Dr. Alessio Fasano, one-third of the population is genetically predisposed to celiac. If 33 percent of Americans are predisposed, why is it still relatively uncommon? Dr. Fasano says:

> "There must be some environmental factors that explain why most people [with the genetic predisposition] eat gluten all their lives and stay healthy, and others lose their tolerance. And it could happen at any time. Some people don't become celiac until they are in their 70s. You're not out of the woods at any age.
>
> "The genome is like a marble block. What it will become in terms of a sculpture depends on the environment. Even if we inherit these genes, they are not always functional or expressed.
>
> "We also know that prevalence is rising and we're in the midst of an epidemic. Based on our study it seems that prevalence has doubled every 15 years in North America. Why? I think it goes back to the microbiome. There are antibiotics, our diet has changed, we travel more. There have been so many changes in the past 50 years."

Despite its rarity, celiac disease is twice as common as Crohn's disease, ulcerative colitis, and cystic fibrosis combined! One of the most alarming things about celiac is that you can be asymptomatic but still have it, as Dr. Fasano mentioned in the excerpt above. That's why some people are not diagnosed until well into adulthood. Untreated celiac disease has been linked in rare instances to an increased risk of certain types of cancers, especially intestinal lymphoma.[179,180]

You have celiac disease for life, but, in some cases, those genes aren't turned on and expressed—until they are.

You have celiac disease for life, but, in some cases, those genes aren't turned on and expressed—until they are.

Currently, there are no drugs to treat celiac disease, and there is no cure. The only way to treat the illness is by removing all gluten from the diet. The good news is people with celiac disease can lead a normal, healthy life by following a completely gluten-free diet.

We'd all be better off going gluten-free. Modern wheat is simply not the same plant that God created for human consumption, and our bodies know that better than we do.

The frightening thing about non-celiac gluten sensitivity and food sensitivities in general is they are not like an overt allergy to peanuts where you have an immediate reaction. Symptoms of food sensitivities are delayed three hours to three days later, so many people don't even realize they have a food sensitivity.

Maybe you don't have a reaction to gluten or maybe you do. If you're consuming multiple foods to which you are sensitive, there is no way you'll ever know.

A patient who was hesitant to give up wheat once said to me, "Jesus is the bread of life, Dani, not the quinoa of life."

> **A patient who was hesitant to give up wheat once said to me, "Jesus is the bread of life, Dani, not the quinoa of life."**

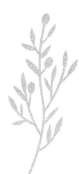

That's both hilarious and true—but Jesus only had three types of wheat when he walked this earth. Modern wheat is an absolute Frankenfood. Don't eat it because of the gluten, and, if you ever get tempted, remember the chemicals used to kill it before it's harvested. Then remember the thyroid dysfunction. Also, don't forget that the glue-like gluten will act like morphine and cause you to crave it more and more. Then remember that, ultimately, processed flour will rob you of health and happiness in the form of gut dysfunction, weight gain, inflammation, and more.

The Bottom Line

Modern wheat is the Frankenstein's monster of the food world. It was created in labs through hybridization. Then it is sprayed with poison, made with indigestible protein that makes many people sick, and infused with toxic chemicals, all so that the bread will be fluffier and cheaper—and more addictive.

DANI'S TIPS FOR SAYING GOODBYE TO GLUTEN

If bread is your kryptonite, I get it.

Lots of my patients have been able to say farewell to added sugars, but when it comes to bread, it's a different story. How can you live without another sandwich or burger for the rest of your life?

I'm not going to sit here and pretend that two pieces of lettuce instead of bread are going to cut it for everyone. So, what I recommend first is to decide that letting go of gluten is important enough to find acceptable alternatives.

In my experience, an open mind always makes food taste better.

Next, focus on finding whole-food-based bread alternatives. The issue to keep in mind is that most of the pre-made, commercial gluten-free breads may contain other ingredients that you would do best to avoid.

For example, one of the most popular and widely available gluten-free bread makers on the market, Udi's Gluten Free, uses eggs and corn syrup solids in their bread recipes. So, while the bread may not contain gluten, I certainly wouldn't call it "healthy."

If you can't live without bread, your best bet is to make your own gluten-free bread at home with brown rice, almond, cassava, or coconut flours. That way you can still enjoy a sandwich from time to time or a burger without the gluten.

However, I'd like to add that time and time again, I've seen patients who were unable to shed pounds after switching to gluten-free breads.

I don't wish to be the bearer of bad news here, but eating bread every day, glutenous or otherwise, is not going to get you where you need to be. Bread made with other grains could also be inflammatory for you, and breads made with nut flour are calorically dense.

Give your body a break *and* a fighting chance and explore new ways to treat yourself and indulge. Reserve gluten-free bread consumption for date nights or special nights out with friends. For the rest of the time, make filling, satisfying homemade meals filled with clean protein, fat, and veggies—and just say no to breads. There are resources in the back of this book for you to learn more about gluten and how to eat a simple one-ingredient food diet with no gluten. There's also a list of hidden places where gluten is found, such as soy sauce, salad dressings, soups, and so much more.

Going gluten free is a positive and impressive first step in the right direction, but it can't stop there. Let's take the next step into the magical but highly inflammatory land of milk and cheese.

The Difficulty with Dairy

2. Once upon a time, many ages ago, someone saw a calf sipping milk from his mother's udder and thought, "I'd like to get in on that action."

Since that day, we've been downing milk and eating products made from milk—a liquid that is produced by a cow to feed its young.

We are the only mammals on earth who drink the milk of another mammal, and we are the only mammals who drink milk of *any* kind into adulthood. Of course, we are also the only species who use toilets, cook meals, write books, and drive cars. So, that fact alone doesn't necessarily mean milk is not intended for human consumption.

Still, with so much circulating in the news about the dangers of dairy, should we assume that mankind was never meant to drink milk? Just like with bread and wheat, the issue is not that clear cut. Humans are set apart from the rest of the animal kingdom in many ways. According to the Bible, there is nothing wrong with milk consumption.

Milk is mentioned in the ancient text in numerous places, and it is understood that God gave us cows as a food source. In the book of Exodus, the Lord said to Moses and his brother Aaron:

> "Speak to the people of Israel, saying, 'These are the living things that you may eat among all the animals that are on the earth. Whatever parts the hoof and is cloven-footed and chews the cud, among the animals, you may eat.'"

In other words, cud-chewing cows have always been on the menu. One could infer that means their milk always has been, too. In fact, the destination that Moses was leading his people to was referred to by God as a land "flowing with milk and honey."

So, what's the deal with milk?

LACTOSE: THE ORIGINAL MILK ISSUE

When it comes to milk consumption, there are several commonly cited problems. The first and most familiar one is the sugar found in milk, called lactose. As babies, we produce a digestive enzyme called lactase that can break down the lactose in our mother's milk. However, as we age, we are said to lose the ability to break down lactose.[181] Hence, some develop a well-known condition known as lactose intolerance. Studies suggest that around 44 percent of Americans are lactose intolerant.[182]

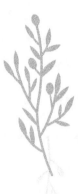

> **A symptom is never just a symptom and nothing more. There is always more under the surface than meets the eye. Where there is smoke, there is FIRE.**

Lactose intolerance is something I've heard about my whole life. Strangely enough, I remember it was always marginalized into being considered an inconvenient and sometimes even *amusing* condition.

"I *love* ice cream, but I know when I eat it, there'll be hell to pay an hour later."

However, the problems with milk consumption surpass a little gas. Lactose intolerance may only manifest as some digestive distress, diarrhea, and bloating, but consider the chronic inflammation that those symptoms may likely represent.

A symptom is never just a symptom and nothing more. There is always more under the surface than meets the eye. Where there is smoke, there is FIRE.

As you may be able to guess, lactose intolerance is linked to low-grade chronic inflammation in human studies.[183]

You know that common notion that milk makes your bones stronger? Yeah, not so much. Milk actually depletes calcium from your bones! Dairy product consumption is associated with an increased risk of hip fracture in old age.[184] In a study of more than 40,000 people with osteoarthritis, researchers determined that patients who regularly consumed dairy were more likely to need hip replacement surgery.[185]

The science behind it is straightforward: Like all animal protein, milk acidifies your body pH. Because your body continually strives for balance and neutral pH, this triggers a biological correction. And, because calcium is such an efficient acid neutralizer, your body uses its calcium stores in your bones to neutralize the acidifying effects of milk! Isn't it ironic?

CASEIN: PROTEIN OR PUBLIC ENEMY?

The next and even bigger issue with dairy is casein. It's one of two proteins found in milk—the other being whey. Casein is a lesser-known inflammatory agent compared to lactose, but it is quickly growing in familiarity thanks to mounting bodies of research on the subject.

I personally have casein, goat's milk, and cow's milk sensitivities. My body has no problem with lactose, but it still hates dairy! That's unfortunate for me, since I love cheese more than any other food on earth.

Interestingly, in studies on the effects of chronic inflammation on the development of metabolic disorders and diabetes, mice were *injected with casein* to induce chronic inflammation! According to the researchers, "Chronic inflammation induced by casein injection further decreased insulin sensitivity and insulin signaling, resulting in insulin deficiency and hyperglycemia."[186]

Casein has also been linked to the development of autoimmune diseases such as Crohn's disease and inflammatory bowel diseases such as ulcerative colitis.[187] I have lupus—and, remember, I spent 44 years on this planet before anyone ever asked me about my diet.

The Awful Truth
Scientists inject animals with casein to induce inflammation in laboratory tests. Let that sink in for a minute.

There are different types of casein, one of which is called beta-casein. Beta-casein makes up about 30 percent of the protein in cow's milk. A1 and A2 are two variants of beta-casein. The structure of A2 protein is more comparable to human breast milk, as well as milk from goats, sheep, and buffalo.

Interest in the difference between A1 and A2 beta-casein proteins began in the early 1990s by some New Zealand scientists who were studying diabetes and heart disease and accidentally discovered an unlikely culprit in disease development. They found shocking correlations between the prevalence of milk with A1 beta-casein proteins and the occurrence of various chronic diseases.[188]

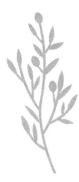

Today, the milk available at grocery stores contains mostly the A1 form of beta-casein.

Many millennia ago (in the days where God's people lived in the land of milk and honey), A2 was the most common variety of milk. Scientists say the now-prevalent A1 variation mutated in Europe as long as 5,000 to 10,000 years ago—but the *why* behind the change is not certain.

Some believe that when farmers started breeding for higher output, they opted for A1-dominant breeds like Holsteins that are known for producing more milk.

Today, the milk available at grocery stores contains mostly the A1 form of beta-casein.

A 2017 study showed that milk containing A1 promoted intestinal inflammation and exacerbated gastrointestinal symptoms.[189] In fact, some researchers now believe that it is a peptide called beta-casomorphin-7 (BCM-7), not lactose, that negatively affects digestion. When A1 protein is digested in the small intestine, it produces BCM-7 that then gets passed into the blood. Doctors have linked BCM-7 to symptoms similar to those experienced by people with lactose intolerance.[190] BCM-7 is also linked in animal studies to the slowing of intestinal motility (movement).[191]

Interestingly, milk containing *only* A2 may not have the same harmful effects as does milk with A1. In the same 2017 study, A2 milk actually *diminished* GI-related symptoms in adults, while A1/A2 milk reduced the body's ability to produce sufficient lactase enzyme and also increased GI-related symptoms.[192]

The A2 variant of casein did not reduce lactase enzyme (the stuff that breaks down lactose) production, while A1 did.

Another study of adults in China with self-reported milk intolerance compared the effects of drinking regular milk that contained A1 and A2 proteins with A2-only milk on intestinal function and inflammation. The participants consumed eight ounces of milk twice a day for two weeks. They reported worse stomach pain after they consumed the regular milk but no change in symptoms after they drank the A2 milk. Participants also reported more frequent and looser-consistency stools while they drank the regular milk. These symptoms did not occur after they consumed the A2 milk.[193]

Could it be, then, that lactose is not the problem?

The real culprit may be A1 casein.

Is it possible to find milk with only A2 casein? It is now, thanks to companies like The a2 Milk Company, which uses cows who have been DNA-tested and proven only to produce milk with the A2 variant. My son Jackson loves milk but has horrible reactions to dairy, so he recently tried some A2 milk from Sprouts. He drank it and had no GI issues at all!

If you can find A2 milk at your local health store, try it and see how you feel— but remember that because it doesn't contain A1 doesn't suddenly make it perfectly healthy.

However, if they start making A2 cheese, I'll be first in line.

COWS: UNWILLING DRUG ADDICTS

Let's put aside what occurs naturally in dairy and talk about what's being added to your dairy. Conventional dairy cows are *pumped* with antibiotics and fed inflammatory grains in a feedlot. In fact, some estimates say that as much as 80 percent of all antibiotics produced by the pharmaceutical industry are used on animals. There are also positive links to antibiotic resistance in feedlot animals and the antibiotic resistance epidemic our nation currently faces.

The antibiotics are just the start. Then there are the hormones. All milk (whether from humans, cows, goats, or dolphins) naturally contains small amounts of various hormones, including estrogen and progesterone. And, despite popular belief, organic milk contains about the same level of hormones as conventionally produced milk.

All milk also contains bovine somatotropin (BST) or bovine growth hormone (BGH), which are naturally occurring hormones in cows that help them produce milk. rBST, a synthetic copy of this hormone, is often given to cows by dairy farmers to boost milk production.

It doesn't stop there. The lactose sugars in dairy stimulate the release of insulin in humans, as well as a hormone called insulin-like growth factor-1 (IGF-1). This is important to note because insulin/IGF-1 signaling is involved in the regulation of many critical functions and malfunctions including fetal growth, T-cell maturation in the thymus, linear growth, pathogenesis of acne, atherosclerosis, diabetes, obesity, cancer, and neurodegenerative diseases.

Truth Bomb

Sure, hormones are added to conventional milk. But don't forget the naturally occurring hormones found in all milk, including organic and raw.

In short, IGF-1 (and by extension, dairy consumption) affects almost every chronic disease we face today. **Of particular concern is the possibility that milk intake during pregnancy adversely affects the early fetal programming of the IGF-1 axis, which will influence health risks later in life.**[194,195,196]

Were we designed to ingest estrogen from cows? Is it safe to assume that estrogen in cow's milk promotes the growth of hormone-sensitive cancers such as breast or ovarian cancer? What about provoking the onset of early puberty in children? These are all fair questions, but the more burning question is this:

Haven't people been drinking milk for millennia?

They have—but, sadly, we can't compare what we do to what our ancestors did. That's an apples-to-oranges comparison.

Our ancestors, and even those living in America in the early 20th century, didn't have cattle who were fed inflammatory, genetically modified grain.

Their livestock was not injected with hormones and steroids. Their cows did not experience painful trauma by being dehorned without the use of anesthetic or pain relief, and their legs were not covered in hock lesions due to being housed for long periods. They didn't get milk from cows who were completely lame and unable to move due to overcrowding.

You're only as good as the diet of the cow who provided the milk you are drinking.

In the case of conventionally raised animals and even some organic livestock, the quality is questionable at best and downright life-threatening at worst.

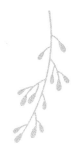

You're only as good as the diet of the cow who provided the milk you are drinking.

THE BOTTOM LINE ON DAIRY

Despite conflicting information, the research presented in the mainstream media paints a pretty picture when it comes to dairy-based products. A 2017 meta-review of 52 clinical studies concluded that dairy "generally has anti-inflammatory effects, except in people allergic to cow's milk." The authors, however, did acknowledge that there is "surprisingly little known about what components of dairy products might be helpful versus harmful."[197]

"It's hard to draw conclusions," says Frank Hu, MD, Ph.D., a professor of epidemiology and nutrition at the Harvard T. H. Chan School of Public Health in Boston. In an article written for the Arthritis Foundation, he explains that it's complicated because the term "dairy" encompasses such a variety of foods. From yogurt and ice cream to milk and cheese—and, of course, all of the variations within each category. Dr. Hu says *that* is why it's so difficult for research to conclusively settle on which components in dairy are good for us and which are not.

I don't know about you, but that is not very comforting to me.

Dairy is a minefield, and it's hard to tell what ingredient (added or otherwise) is causing your inflammation, digestive issues, and other symptoms. I certainly wasn't doing my body any favors by eating those little orange squares that were individually wrapped in plastic when I was a kid. I imagine lots of you did, too—and you may be feeding them to your children today.

You know what the ingredients are in those thin processed quadrangles? It's a lot more than just "cheese" and may include some of the following:

> INGREDIENTS: Natural cheeses or enzyme modified cheeses, emulsifying agents, acidulants (vinegar, lactic acid, citric acid, acetic acid, phosphoric acid), milkfat (from cream, anhydrous milkfat or dehydrated cream), water, salt, colors, spices, flavorings, mold inhibitors (sorbic acid, potassium sorbate, sodium sorbate, and anti-sticking agents.

When you add one of those orange squares to a sandwich, you are eating a food whose *partial* ingredients were sourced from a concrete-bound dairy cow, but that's about the most positive thing I can say about processed cheese products.

Some say that raw milk is better for you. That is true to some extent, since pasteurization destroys enzymes, diminishes vitamin content, kills beneficial bacteria, and promotes pathogens. The process is also associated with allergies, increased tooth decay, colic in infants, growth problems in children, osteoporosis, arthritis, heart disease, and cancer.

So, yes, raw milk is a better choice over processed milk. It's also safe (despite claims on the news) as long as it's properly collected from cows who are fed good, clean grass. However, raw milk still contains A1 casein and lactose, and so if those are inflammatory for you, your problems will persist.

Here is what I *do* know with certainty:

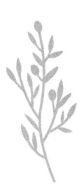

If you've never gone dairy-free, I encourage you to see for yourself how good you will feel without cow pus in your life.

Within a week to ten days of removing *all* dairy from my patients' diets, much of their night-time congestion goes away. Their acne starts to clear, and their eczema calms. Their asthma symptoms begin to decrease. They feel thinner and less bloated, and they experience less brain fog. Their joint pain is diminished. Their seasonal allergy symptoms decrease.

The results speak for themselves. If you've never gone dairy-free, I encourage you to see for yourself how good you will feel without cow pus in your life.

Still, each day I hear the same complaint from patients, which is some variation of, "But do you know how hard it is to cut dairy from my diet?" I sure do! Every time I walk by the cheese section at a grocery store, I immediately want to go taste the Drunken Goat, Manchego, triple soft Brie, and every other cheese from stinky, blue, soft, mild, etc. Then I tell myself, "It's simply cow pus and cow snot, Dani. Back away from the cheese section."

It takes a lot of effort, for sure. Making things more complicated is the fact that our kids are hooked on dairy, too. Most kids I know would gladly live on grilled cheese, mac and cheese, ham and cheese, milk, yogurt, and cheese sticks if they could.

Parents often say to me, "But Dani! My kids just won't stop sneaking into the fridge and eating string cheese!"

> **Stop buying dairy and bringing it home! If it's in the house, it will get eaten.**

My reply is always the same. "How did that string cheese even get into the house? Did your seven-year-old call an Uber for a quick cheese run?"

Stop buying dairy and bringing it home! If it's in the house, it will get eaten.

If you want to keep eating dairy and feeding it to your kids because "that's all they will eat," then I'm certainly not going to judge you. It took me seven long years AFTER I discovered that my body doesn't like dairy to cut it out completely.

> **If you wouldn't give your kids hormones injections, why would you feed them *any* dairy— organic, raw, or otherwise?**

If you aren't ready to make the cut, you can start by making smart choices like opting for A2 milk and using products sourced only from 100 percent pasture-raised cattle. Just keep in mind that A2 milk is likely still pasteurized and may be from cows given antibiotics and GMO grains and confined to concrete prisons. Also, raw milk may contain A1 casein, lactose, and hormones and, depending on the dairy farm, may even contain antibiotics, steroids, and added hormones.

If you are unwilling even to entertain the idea of giving up dairy, you can find whatever study you need to justify how you feel. But the truth doesn't hide. We are sick and bloated and congested. We are chronically inflamed. Our children are reaching puberty sooner than ever.

If you wouldn't give your kids hormones injections, why would you feed them *any* dairy—organic, raw, or otherwise?

Dairy is simply not what it once was. Giving up dairy won't be easy, but I know you can do it. Make the Wild & Well choice and let dairy go.

Crafty Corn

3. The corn sales and marketing people have been putting in some serious overtime hours and are due for a much-needed vacation—and, boy, do they deserve some R&R for a job well done!

Why? Because corn is in EVERYTHING today. Well done, guys.

It's in our food: cereals and snack foods of every shape, size, and flavor; salad dressings; cheese; milk; cough drops; candy; natural supplements; yogurt; desserts; soft drinks; chewing gum; peanut butter; grits; flours; and more.

It's in our non-food: toothpaste, soaps, aspirin, medications, shampoo, dish detergent, diapers, paints, plastic food containers, to-go coffee cups, carpet, adhesives, corks, crayons, linoleum, polish, adhesives, rubber substitutes, batteries, make-up and beauty products, perfumes, candles, dyes, pharmaceuticals, lubricants, insulation, wallpaper, fuel ethanol, industrial enzymes, fuel octane enhancers, and solvents.

> **Haven't we always eaten corn? Sure, we have. The corn of today, however, is just plain nasty.**

Then, then corn they use for biofuel is the very same corn they feed our animals: the distiller's dried grain, gluten feed and meal, and high-oil feed corn for cattle, swine, poultry, and fish.

Even if you diligently avoid all packaged foods and stick with whole fruits, vegetables, and animal products, corn will sneak into your diet. It's gotten completely out of hand. Read that line again… and let it soak in.

Until the 1800s, corn was primarily eaten by the poor. Today, our food has been taken over by this one plant.

Haven't we always eaten corn? Sure, we have. The corn of today, however, is just plain nasty.

When I say "nasty," I am not just being dramatic. Corn is known to contain *aflatoxins*, which are extremely toxic chemicals produced by two molds, Aspergillus parasiticus and Aspergillus flavus. They are often found on agricultural crops such as maize (corn), peanuts, cottonseed, and tree nuts.

Aflatoxin accumulation is usually associated with poor storage conditions. However, hot, dry conditions during grain fill increase the risk of Aspergillus infection and aflatoxin contamination in the field.

Aflatoxins are bad news. They cause DNA mutations and increase your risk of developing cancer cells.[198] The International Food Policy Research Institute reports that "consumption of even tiny amounts of aflatoxin can have a cumulative effect, and can lead to liver damage, gastrointestinal dysfunction, decreased appetite, decreased reproductive function, and decreased growth."[199]

Corn containing less than 20 parts per billion aflatoxin is considered safe by the U.S. Food and Drug Administration for use in animal feed. That may seem like a miniscule amount, but if corn tests too high, it must simply be blended with less toxic corn before serving up the mold to our animals. Making matters more complex is the fact that the standards only apply to corn that crosses state lines. If the food is produced in the same state where it's being used, well, too bad.

And, according to Fox News, "actual aflatoxin concentration in animal feed may at times be higher" due to the lack of standardized federal inspection.

Yikes.

So maybe *you* aren't eating moldy corn—but the dairy and feedlot cows are, and the chickens and turkeys are, and the pigs are. That's why, if you're going to eat meat and animal products, those animals should not be fed a grain-rich diet.

Even if it's a seemingly insignificant part of the animal's diet, the corn can be enough to trigger inflammation and an immune response in YOU when you eat that gluten-free hamburger or have your daily yogurt.

You may think you are gluten and corn free, but if your animal isn't, then neither are you.

GM-OH NO!

Have you ever witnessed or even seen a picture of an animal in the wild munching on stalks of corn? No! Cows eat grass. Chickens eat all kinds of things including wild seeds, worms, insects, berries, fruits, and nuts.

Notice that list does not include moldy, genetically engineered corn.

These trials are conducted in secret by the GMO-associated companies who profit when the tests show no adverse results.

Genetic modification is a controversial topic. Currently in the U.S., GM crops make up to 94 percent of planted acres for corn, soybeans, and cotton. Plenty of scientists claim that foods made with genetically modified seeds are perfectly healthy. However, common sense would tell you otherwise.

Peer-reviewed journal *Environment International* noted back in 2011 that a large number of research groups have reported many varieties of GM products (particularly corn and soy) to be "as safe and nutritious as the respective conventional non-GM plant." But then the authors added this important line:

> "Nevertheless, it should be noted that most of these studies have been conducted by biotechnology companies responsible of commercializing these GM plants."

I don't know about you, but I'm far too awake to blindly believe the studies funded by those who profit *most* from GM foods.

Every time a new gene is inserted into a food to create a novel strain that is more resistant to various poisons or grows more quickly, there is little research done to determine how that gene will affect humans before it is commercialized and sold. The safety "research" done on GMOs is said to involve a three-month feeding trial on lab rats.

These trials are conducted in secret by the GMO-associated companies who profit when the tests show no adverse results.

In 2019, Health and Biotechnology Biopharma reported that, "Contrary to the present biotechnological claims, transgenic products have not proved to be harmless and in many in vivo studies have shown harmful effects."[200]

GMOs are likely causing untold damage to us through direct ingestion and indirect ingestion of animals who were fed GMOs. So, is there any corn that is good for you? It's disappearing rapidly, but if you can find *heirloom corn* and don't have a sensitivity to corn according to food testing, that may be a viable option. There are still around 200 varieties of heirloom corn available, and they come in a rainbow of vibrant colors (forget that sad, pale yellow you see in the grocery store).

THE CRISIS INTENSIFIES

I predict that as the gluten-free diet continues its meteoric rise in popularity, more and more people will develop adverse reactions to corn. That's because corn is the go-to grain used in place of wheat in many of those processed, gluten-free man-made packaged foods.

And don't even get me started on high-fructose corn syrup.

High-fructose corn syrup is cheap and stable... and destroying our health.

High-fructose corn syrup is a cheap, highly stable liquid sweetener found in countless processed foods. Sometimes companies even claim that their products are "natural" even though they contain high-fructose corn syrup. According to researchers at North Carolina Central University, the increase in the consumption of high-fructose corn syrup "has coincided with the increase in incidence of obesity, heart disease, and other cardiovascular diseases and metabolic syndromes."[201]

If you're eating processed foods, you've got to look on the back of the package, and you've got to know all the names for corn.

And there are a ton.

Lastly, remember this: When factory farms want to fatten up cows and pigs quickly, what do they feed them? Corn. While plenty of people think of corn as a vegetable, it's really just another inflammatory grain.

If you want to get fattened up and sick in a hurry, corn is the way to go. But no Wild & Well believer wants that, so read labels, or, better yet, eat single-ingredient foods.

Names for Corn on Food Labels

- Corn syrup/high fructose corn syrup
- Sucrose (used to be from cane sugar, but now often corn)
- Fructose, glucose
- Maltodextrin, dextrin
- Dextrose
- Sorbitol
- Malt, malt syrup, malt extract
- Excipients (a binder in pills)
- Glucona delta lactone or GDL (found in cured meats)
- Monoglycerides, diglycerides
- Mono-Sodium Glutamate (MSG) is often corn-derived
- Sugar (if it doesn't say beet or cane)
- Corn starch, starch, modified food starch
- Carmel flavoring or coloring (made from corn syrup)
- Vegetable oil, vegetable broth, vegetable protein
- Hydrolyzed vegetable protein, vegetable mono- or diglycerides.
- Xanthan gum (a thickener often grown in corn media)
- Zein (a fiber made from corn)

Soy the Insidious

When it comes to life-threatening food allergies (the kind that can land you in the ER or worse), most people think of foods like shellfish and peanuts. Although it's one of the less talked about allergies, soy should certainly be on everyone's radar. From hives and swelling to wheezing and anaphylactic shock, a soy allergy is nothing to sneeze at.

Even if you aren't allergic to soy, just like with dairy and gluten, being *sensitive* to soy manifests in the form of unpleasant yet ambiguous symptoms such as eczema, acne, breathing issues, sinusitis, digestive symptoms including nausea and diarrhea, canker sores, and colitis.

Did you notice those "itis" words in there? Yep, soy is yet another food that is linked to inflammation.

Still—and this may be a bit controversial—I don't believe soy is the devil. If it were, then the life expectancy in Japan wouldn't be so high. Japan comes in at number two on the world's life expectancy ranking, and yet they eat soy for breakfast, lunch, and dinner.

Japanese eat more soybeans than anyone else, and the famed long-life-prone Okinawans top the list of soy consumption at about 60 to 120 grams per person each day.

Before you assume that all the Japanese are eating is fermented forms of soy, think again. In Japan, about half of soy intake comes from fermented foods such as natto and miso—and the rest is tofu. They also enjoy whole bean edamame and fresh soy milk.

So, what gives? It once again goes back not to the food itself but to modern farming and food manufacturing. Ancient wheat and corn were once nutritious. Now they are two of the primary culprits behind obesity and escalating rates of disease. People have been drinking dairy since the beginning, and yet now so many are sensitive to it.

See the pattern here? Soy follows it, too.

There are the traditional ways to eat soy (such as making tofu and fermenting the soy), and then there are the mad-scientist-type methods of processing soy, and we eat the results every day. Food manufacturers isolate the protein and use the by-product, known as soy isoflavone, as an additive.

Michael Pollan, author of the incredible book, *In Defense of Food: An Eater's Manifesto*, says that 20 percent of the American diet now comes from soy or soy oil. Did you know you were eating that much soy? Of course you didn't.

> **Soy is in nearly 75 percent of products in the grocery store and in nearly 100 percent of fast food.**

My patients who have a soy allergy or sensitivity tell me all the time how difficult it is to buy, well, virtually *anything*, since soy is lurking all around us. Soybeans—which are legumes that are related to clover, peas, and alfalfa—are incredibly versatile as a food, but, like corn, soy is also used in thousands of products such as soaps, cosmetics, plastics, clothing, inks, glues, lubricants, coatings, and insulation. It's even in your SUPPLEMENTS!

Raj Patel, author of *Stuffed & Starving* reports that:

Soy is in nearly 75 percent of products in the grocery store and in nearly 100 percent of fast food.

It's all starting to make sense. The Asian cultures may be eating soy, but they are eating whole legumes, fresh tofu, soy milk, and fermented soy while we are eating rancid soybean oil and processed foods stuffed with cheap, genetically modified soy derivatives.

Did You Know?

Soy lecithin is found in so many foods! It's used as an emulsifier (makes water and oil mix), a surfactant (a wetting agent), an anti-stick and anti-foaming agent, and a shelf-life extender. You will be hard-pressed to find a product in the grocery store without this ingredient listed.

Every packaged, processed packet and bottle you pick up in the grocery store probably has some derivative of soy in it—and the vegan craze is only making things worse! Don't believe me? Here is a great example of what I mean:

Instead of eating a healing, anti-inflammatory fat such as pasture-raised, organic clarified butter (ghee), more and more people are opting for vegan butters. Here are the ingredients of one of the most popular and widespread vegan butters called Earth Balance (and this is the organic version):

> INGREDIENTS: Vegetable Oil Blend (Palm Fruit, Soybean, Canola, Olive Oils), Water, Salt, Contains Less Than 2% Of Natural Flavor, Defatted Soy Flour, Soy Lecithin, Lactic Acid (To Protect Freshness), Annatto Extract (Color).

Compare that to the ingredients of grass-fed ghee, whose label lists just a single ingredient:

> INGREDIENTS: Certified organic butter.

The clarification process of the ghee removes the casein and all that remains is a healthy fat, as opposed to the added colors and "natural" flavors added to the soy flour and variety of processed oils in the vegan butter.

Guys, it's time to wake up and make some changes. Quite simply, the safety of consuming huge amounts of highly processed soy is questionable at best.

HORMONE RUSSIAN ROULETTE

The reason why high soy intake is such a potential problem is largely due to hormones. For those of you who may not know, our hormones do more than control our moods or affect our reproductive system and puberty.

Hormones control it all! They are the body's messengers, and they function 24/7 across all systems. It's not a good idea to mess with them or their balance in our bodies.

Phytoestrogens are natural plant compounds abundantly found in soy and soy products that mimic estrogen and are therefore considered endocrine disrupting compounds (EDCs). EDCs alter normal hormone function and cause potentially adverse health effects. While phytoestrogens were once associated with healthy side effects, they are now linked to the possible growth of certain cancers, menopause-like symptoms, and widespread endocrine system dysfunction.

Author Michael Pollan also points out in his book that because of the uncertainties related to the estrogen-mimicking power of phytoestrogens, the FDA has declined to grant GRAS ('generally regarded as safe') status to soy isoflavones used as a food additive.

If the government won't even endorse it—now that's saying something.

If the government won't even endorse it—now that's saying something.

If you are not sensitive to soy and want to include it as a part of your plant-based diet, I encourage you to skip the processed vegan foods with soy as the protein source and consider trying whole-food-based soy products and especially fermented soy products such as natto. While natto can be challenging at first bite due to a unique consistency, it's one of the world's best sources of vitamin K2, which is a bone and heart power-house. Thanks to the modern diet, the average intake of this key nutrient is shockingly low.

I fully realize that soy is an essential element of most plant-based diets. I'm not telling you *not* to go plant-based, but I will say that, like it or not, soy will affect your hormone levels in some way. Will that lead to inflammation or disease?

No one can say with precise certainty.

NYrture New York Natto is a popular brand of natto that is made right here in the U.S. It's a living fermented food that packs a powerful nutritional punch! Check them out at: **NYrture.com**

Sugar is For Suckers

5. In case you haven't been paying attention to any news for the last few decades, let's just say that conventional practitioners and holistic professionals alike are all in agreement that sugar is bad.

Just 200 years ago, the average American only ate two pounds of sugar a year. By 1970, we were up to 123 pounds of sugar. Today, the average American consumes almost 152 pounds of sugar in one year. That is equal to three pounds or six cups of sugar consumed in one week.

Pick up a three-pound weight and hold that in your hand. Now picture pouring six entire cups of sugar down your throat every single week, month after month. That is our reality in this country—and it's killing us.

Sugar is linked to the development of every chronic lifestyle disease we face today.

There are plausible mechanisms and research evidence that supports the sug-

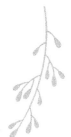

Sugar is linked to the development of every chronic lifestyle disease we face today.

gestion that consumption of excess sugar promotes the development of cardiovascular disease and type 2 diabetes both directly and indirectly.[202] You have no doubt heard that obesity is linked to heart disease and type 2 diabetes—and, as you can easily guess, sugar intake and obesity are positively correlated.[203]

Shocking But True
The average person eats 152 pounds of sugar a year.

But what is more surprising for some is that a sugar-laden diet may raise your risk of dying of heart disease even if you aren't overweight, according to a major study published in *JAMA Internal Medicine*.[204]

You are not born obese or with type 2 diabetes. Most of us are not born with autoimmune disease. We eat the things that cause chronic inflammation, and that inflammation starts a cascade of events inside your body that lead to more problems and, eventually, pain and sickness. Decades of dysfunction turn on chronic disease.

Sugar also affects your temperament and outlook on life. In a study on the effects of sugar on energy and mood, researchers asked one group of people to take a short walk, while another group reached for a sugary snack instead of going for a walk. As you may be able to predict, "walking was associated with higher self-rated energy and lower tension significantly more than was snacking." Snacking on sugary foods was associated with significantly higher tension after just one hour, not to mention a vicious pattern of initially increased energy followed by increased tiredness and reduced energy.[205]

We are not the only nation to be paying a heavy price (literally and figuratively) for our love of sweetness. The obesity and chronic disease epidemics currently ongoing in America have spread to every country where sugar-based carbohydrates have come to dominate to the food economy.[206]

If God created sugar, why is it so harmful? At the risk of sounding like a broken record, here goes: It is *modern* sugar and all of its various, *processed* forms that are the problem. (Well, that and sheer quantity. We are obsessed!)

Once upon a time, the human diet contained very little sugar and virtually no refined carbohydrates.[207] Some say that sugar may have even been introduced into our diets by accident. The common understanding is that for most of history, sugarcane was used as a "fodder" crop for fattening up livestock.

At some point, however, sugar started to work its addictive magic on us, and the rest, as they say, is history. Sugar granules were invented around 2,000 years ago. Since then, humans have been getting really creative with sugar production and eventually expanded into the development of addictive, super sweet sugars like beet sugar and high-fructose corn syrup.

Amazingly, sugar was once considered a fine spice and was priced too high for everyone except the ultra-wealthy. Today, you can walk into any grocery store and buy pounds and pounds of it for pennies.

It's almost as though they *want* us to be sick and fat.

UBIQUITOUS AND ADDICTIVE

Sugar—a food (I use that term loosely) that has no nutritional value and provides an inferior source of energy—had a hand in directing the formation of the Americas as we know them. The demand for labor at the massive sugar plantations, along with the tobacco plantations, in Brazil and the Caribbean is a huge part of what drove the transatlantic slave trade.

Both products were once considered to be good for us—and maybe at one point in history, some ancient form of sugar was. In fact, there is evidence that sugarcane was used for medicinal purposes in Ancient Rome and Greece.

Ever seen one of those old ads for cigarettes with doctors in lab coats singing tobacco's praises? Similar ads exist for sugar! As consumers, we tend to believe whatever our magazines and newspapers tell us, andbelieve me, advertisers know this.

Wow. Just… wow.

Today, we know the truth. Sugar is as addictive as heroin and cocaine, and possibly even more destructive since it's perfectly legal and available everywhere without any stigmas attached.

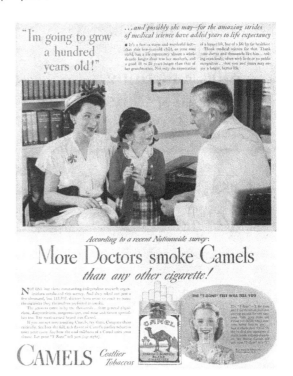

In fact, having a sugar addiction is laughed off as being inevitable, as in, "My son has a sweet tooth just like his dad." Everyone just shrugs and laughs and keeping stuffing their faces with Ding Dongs.

Sugar is like corn and soy—it's everywhere! Added sugar is the most prevalent ingredient added to foods in the U.S. When you read a label, sugar will probably be there in some form. Added sugar is found in cakes, cookies, yogurt, candy, ketchup, crackers, bread, soup, cereal, peanut butter, "healthy" smoothies, energy drinks, cured meat, salad dressing, and so much more. And yet, the recommended amount of sugar intake is as follows:

Men: 150 calories per day (37.5 grams or 9 teaspoons)
Women: 100 calories per day (25 grams or 6 teaspoons)

Folks, that's *not* a lot of sugar.

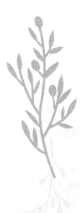

> "A fruit is a vegetable with looks and money. Plus, if you let fruit rot, it turns into wine, something Brussels sprouts never do."
>
> P. J. O'ROURKE

Considering one soda has anywhere from 7 to 11 teaspoons and your average energy drink has up to 17 teaspoons of sugar, those numbers are easy to surpass by breakfast. A plain ole Starbucks Grande Latte (not even a Venti mocha or peppermint) has your entire allotment of sugar (25 grams) in one little cup.

Another alarming trend that is affecting even the health-conscious is the widespread acceptance of daily wine drinking. Daily wine consumption has become so common and accepted as a nightly ritual and even seen as a status symbol on social media. While wine (particularly red wine) does have numerous health benefits, the problem is that lots of wineries actually *add* sugar to their wine, taking a beverage that is rich in antioxidants and loading it with unnecessary sugar and calories.

If you are going to drink wine, you better make sure it's clean-crafted wine that comes from non-GMO vineyards that don't add sugar to their products. My go-to wines of choice are labels through Scout and Cellar, who make clean-crafted wines with no added sugar, no pesticides, and no other added

CLEAN-CRAFTED WINE

* Grapes
* Usually less than 50ppm of sulfites*

Always less than 100ppm

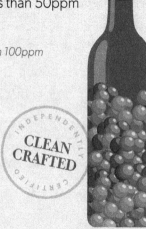

CLEAN CRAFTED

MASS-PRODUCED WINE

* Grapes
* Up to 350ppm of sulfites
* Up to 16g of added sugar or sweetener concentrate
* Ferrocyanide
* Ammonium phosphate
* Copper sulfate
* Mega-Purple
* GMO ingredients
* Synthetic pesticides

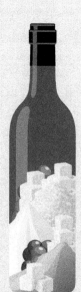

garbage. See the resource section in the back for a link to learn about what's in your wine and how to get clean-crafted wine that is organic, safe, no added sugar, and low in sulfites.

If you are struggling to lose weight, you may want to look at your wine intake. One of my patients lost 15 pounds in just two months without changing *anything* other than one thing—she stopped drinking wine. It's a step that is worth considering if you can't seem to shake the weight.

DANI'S TIPS FOR SAYING 'SO LONG!' TO SUGAR

I am here to tell you that cutting out gluten and dairy was much easier for me than removing sugar. After every single meal, I want something sweet. Anything. And frozen grapes don't do the trick for me.

It's a daily struggle, but I wake up every day and fight the good fight because it's too important.

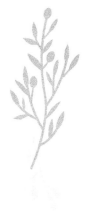

If you are committed to giving up sugar, give yourself a pat on the back! But don't expect sugar to give up without a struggle. Be ready to face some withdrawal symptoms because sugar is proven to be addictive. Animal data has shown significant overlap between the consumption of added sugars and drug-like effects, including bingeing, craving, tolerance, withdrawal, cross-sensitization, cross-tolerance, cross-dependence, reward, and opioid effects.[208]

We keep coming back because we want the high that we feel from the natural opioids that get released upon sugar intake.

We keep coming back because we want the high that we feel from the natural opioids that get released upon sugar intake.

If you want some help, here are some ideas for weaning off the bad stuff:

1. Stop buying it! Step one is to stop bringing cookies and cakes and candies into the house. If it's there, it will get eaten. When your cravings start talking, don't make it easy to reach into the pantry to satisfy them. Your family may protest at first, but this decision is as much about their health and their future as it is about your health journey. If you shouldn't eat it, neither should your kids. Take control of your family's sweet tooth while you still have an influence over them and their decisions, and help make their future brighter by eliminating their own sugar addictions.

2. **Embrace fruit.** While fruit contains sugar in the form of fructose, the amount of fructose is considerably lower than the sugar content of most sweets with added sugar. Even better, according to the WHO, sugars naturally occurring in fruit (but NOT fruit juice) don't count toward that 25-gram daily allotment. Added sugar is the real devil here. So, if fruit satisfies your sweet tooth, then indulge in some berries after dinner. The darker the better.

3. **Dress up your berries.** For those of you who aren't satisfied with just fruit (that's me), then treat yourself to a small scoop of non-dairy cool whip (Cocowhip by So Delicious is my all-time favorite and has just 2 grams of sugar per serving!) and a few shavings of dark chocolate on top. Just be aware of serving sizes and don't eat the whole container. ALWAYS measure.

4. **Use satisfying alternatives.** Stevia, monk fruit, and erythritol are three sweet alternatives to sugar that have no calories and minimal to no effect on blood sugar. There are loads of recipes for treats that contain these healthier alternatives. However, a word of caution is in order: Moderation is the key when it comes to sugar alternatives, especially since these natural sugar substitutes have been known to cause digestive upset in some people. So, you may or may not be able to stomach them. Experiment with these in small doses to assess your tolerance.

Sugar by the Serving

One average candy bar: 35 grams

One average bakery cupcake: 34 grams

Two average cookies: 15 grams

One medium banana: 14 grams

One extra dark (88%) chocolate bar: 9 grams

One cup of strawberries: 7 grams

One cup of raspberries: 5 grams

5. **Get out of the nightly habit.** If you want to have a nightly bowl of berries, go for it. However, I recommend no more than one or two desserts each week sweetened with sugar alternatives. In my experience, conditioning yourself to expect a baked dessert every night is just asking for issues down the road. Train your taste buds to consider heavy desserts to be a special privilege, not a nightly entitlement. Don't forget that baked goodies, even those made with a sugar substitute, are typically high in calories and carbohydrates and could therefore lead to weight gain or inhibit weight loss.

6. **Chew some gum.** Gum brands such as Pur, Spry, and Thrive make great tasting gum that can satisfy the need for something sweet and are also good for your teeth. They are sweetened with xylitol, which is a natural sweetener that has a lower glycemic impact than sugar but still packs a sweet punch and is also shown to promote healthy teeth by fighting the bacteria that cause cavities. It's important to note that too much xylitol can cause loose stools, so chew in moderation.

7. **Add a few sweet drops to your coffee.** A few drops of stevia in your daily coffee can help satisfy a sweet tooth and keep you away from the office donut tray.

8. **Stir up some gelatin.** Stay away from sugar-free Jell-O because it contains artificial sugar in the form of aspartame. Aspartame has been linked to certain cancers, including non-Hodgkin lymphoma,[209] as well as an increased risk of heart disease.[210] However, the good news is there are some Jell-O substitutes on the market that make a great sugar-free, low calorie treat! The brand Simply Delish makes a great tasting gelatin dessert that is sweetened with erythritol and stevia. It contains zero grams of added sugar, has just six calories per serving, and hardens in less than an hour! At $2.50 per box, it's more expensive than Jell-O but still an affordable sweet treat when eaten on occasion.

9. **Keep your purse or bag stocked.** If you are out and about and hunger strikes, make sure to have something on hand to pop in your mouth. I recommend a small handful of nuts or a Lara Bar (contains only nuts and dried fruit). Hunger can cause you to make really dubious choices. So, stock

your car or bag with hunger-thwarting treats and steer clear of the Krispy Kreme drive-through.

10. **Consider a ten-day detox.** I recommend that all of my patients do a thorough detox two to four times a year. During this time, you eliminate added sugars, which works beautifully to stop sugar cravings. There are over 25 years of research on the power of detoxing, and it's proven to decrease inflammation. *You can see my videos on doing a ten-day detox on our YouTube channel.*

Cut out the sugar and see how much better your kids do in school and in interactions with their friends and teachers.

Remove the sugar and discover how much more energy you can have during your usual afternoon crash hours.

Stop the sugar and sleep better.

End your obsession with sugar and finally get control over your mood swings.

Heal from your sugar addiction and lose weight and start eliminating disease markers from your life!

Polluted Peanuts

6.

You are probably not surprised to see peanuts on this list. For me, it's heartbreaking. There is almost nothing in this world I love more than a giant spoonful of Jif brand peanut butter, straight from the jar. I could eat a peanut butter and jelly sandwich every day for the rest of my life and never tire of it.

It's inexpensive and satisfying and good.

But believe me, I'd never say that within 100 feet of a school building, or some alarms might start going off at the mere mention of peanuts.

For those of us with children, we know that peanut allergies plague the schools at epidemic levels. Daycares and schools across the country are becoming peanut-free zones in order to protect those children with life-threatening allergies. You can't even get peanuts on flights anymore.

When did the peanut become public enemy #1?

That's a complicated question with complicated answers. For now, let's focus on some facts about peanuts that can't be disputed.

First, a peanut is not actually a nut. Most nuts are technically considered fruits, but because peanuts grow in the ground (instead of on trees and bushes like other nuts), they are legumes, which are technically vegetables. So, when people have allergies to peanuts, they may or may not have allergies to tree nuts, since the two are quite different.

When did the peanut become public enemy #1?

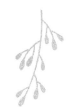

To get even more technical, peanuts are little seeds inside pods and are more closely related to soybeans, chickpeas, peas, clover, licorice, and lentils than nuts.

The fact that peanuts grow on the ground instead of on a bush or tree is one of the reasons why they are so inflammatory. About 75 percent of all cropland in the U.S. is annually sprayed with more than a *billion* pounds of chemicals on crops, including the herbicide glyphosate, also known by its most famous branded name, Roundup.

The carcinogenic and inflammatory effects of herbicides such as glyphosate are well established. Given that, would you be surprised to learn that there are *no* government agencies that monitor risks to farmworkers who labor among those chemicals—or to pregnant women and children who live near agricultural fields?

To combat the damaging effects of chemicals on our crops, the Environmental Working Group (EWG) started publishing a list of the cleanest and most contaminated crops each year. They call it the Dirty Dozen and the Clean Fifteen. Turn to the following page for the most recent version of that list (and go to EWG.org for loads of research on everything from food to beauty products).

While peanuts aren't listed, I'm including this list here because it's important to know which crops are essential to buy organic. And I believe that because peanuts grow in the ground, it should be a food that you *always* buy organic (if your body tolerates the faux nut, that is).

ewg's *dirty dozen*™

1. STRAWBERRIES	5. APPLES	9. PEARS
2. SPINACH	6. GRAPES	10. TOMATOES
3. KALE	7. PEACHES	11. CELERY
4. NECTARINES	8. CHERRIES	12. POTATOES

ewg's *clean fifteen*™

1. AVOCADO	6. SWEET PEAS	11. BROCCOLI
2. SWEET CORN	7. EGGPLANT	12. MUSHROOMS
3. PINEAPPLE	8. ASPARAGUS	13. CABBAGE
4. ONIONS	9. CAULIFLOWER	14. HONEYDEW
5. PAPAYA	10. CANTALOUPE	15. KIWI

Each list is updated yearly. Go to EWG.org/foodnews for the most up-to-date lists.

One particularly alarming detail is the price disparity between organic and conventionally grown fruits and veggies. For example, organic strawberries at the grocery store are often double or even triple the price in some seasons! That forces many of us to buy conventional and wash them thoroughly—and then just hope for the best. The problem is, conventionally grown strawberries are the number one chemically laden offender for the last four years.

Spinach is another major toxic food, with more pesticides by weight than any other crop. A neurotoxic insecticide called permethrin is also found on spinach—and that's a problem because it's linked to ADHD.[211]

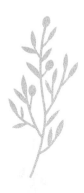

> **We're feeding our kids spinach, thinking we are making healthy choices for them, only to learn that we are contributing to the ADHD epidemic among our children.**

We're feeding our kids spinach, thinking we are making healthy choices for them, only to learn that we are contributing to the ADHD epidemic among our children.

Plenty of parents think that peanuts are a good choice for their kids, too. Peanut butter is cheap, some brands are low in sugar, and it provides a decent amount of protein without much sugar. What's not to love?

Unfortunately, as you are now beginning to see—a lot.

Aside from the pesticides, there is also the mold to consider. Like corn, peanuts are known to contain aflatoxin, the carcinogen that's especially toxic to the liver. It's just another problem with them being grown in the ground—they are grown in darkness and dampness and therefore extremely prone to mold.

Not everybody has a peanut allergy or even a sensitivity, but I advise that all patients eliminate peanuts for at least three weeks. You may not be sensitive to peanuts, but your body definitely doesn't like the mold and pesticides.

If you plan to eat peanuts or feed them to your family in some form, I recommend consuming only Valencia peanuts and peanut butter made with Valencia peanuts to avoid the pesticides and mold issues. Also, make sure to choose organic, because pesticides aren't just inflammatory and carcinogenic—they are also hormone disrupters. Over one-quarter of conventional peanut butter samples tested positive for a known hormone-disrupting pesticide.

For those of you who are near a Trader Joe's, their brand of organic peanut butter is made with Valencia peanuts, and there are only two ingredients: Organic Valencia peanuts and sea salt. The Kirkland brand sold at Costco also makes an organic peanut butter made with Valencia peanuts.

Why are Valencia Peanuts Better?

Peanut butter made from Valencia peanuts has the least amount of aflatoxin on the market. They come from a dry climate (almost exclusively New Mexico) where they are less susceptible to mold growth.

You can enjoy an apple with peanut butter again, as long as peanuts are not on your food sensitivity list. However, as with all of our other food choices, remember that even organic Valencia peanuts will still cause inflammation if you are sensitive to peanuts in any way. So, remove them from your diet for at least three weeks and when you add them back in, note any changes and new symptoms, including GI distress and mood changes.

Not So Extraordinary Eggs

7. To finish our Sinister Seven discussion, we're going to talk about one of the most perfect foods on the planet—the egg. Cheap, versatile, and delicious, it is loaded with tons of vitamins, minerals, and choline.

If you have tried keto, a Whole 30 diet, or the Paleo lifestyle, there is no doubt that eggs have been a huge part of your life. Egg nutrition is impressive, and it provides a sense of fullness and satisfaction like almost nothing else can. It's the perfect breakfast food. It's a flawless low-carb snack. Deviled eggs are an awesome appetizer.

What's not to love?

Little Known Fact

After cow's milk, hen's egg allergy is the second most common food allergy in infants and young children.

Sadly, I rarely eat them anymore because they are on my food sensitivity list, a trait I have in common with *many* other people.

Some react to the proteins in the yolk, some to the proteins in egg whites, and some to both. I react to both the yolk and the albumin (egg white). In general, however, most people who have an egg allergy are allergic to either the ovomucoid or the ovalbumin (also called albumin) in the egg white. The majority of egg-intolerant people tend to be okay with the egg yolk, but it's the egg white, or albumin, that their bodies can't handle. And, because it's not possible to ever fully separate the egg from the yolk, that means no portion of the egg is okay to eat for those with an allergy or sensitivity to any part of an egg.

If you don't have an egg allergy, could you still have an egg intolerance? You bet. The most common symptoms are gastrointestinal in nature and include gas, bloating, and diarrhea, which are pretty much the same intolerance symptoms for the other six foods in this chapter.

Therefore, it's impossible to know for sure if your body doesn't like eggs unless you remove *all* potential inflammatory foods and slowly reintroduce them one at a time or have a high-quality food sensitivity test done.

We can safely assume people have been eating eggs since the first hens started clucking. So, what the problem now?

First, chickens are no longer fed what chickens were designed to eat or even allowed access to sunshine. Thanks to modern farming, conventional chickens are fed an all-grain-based diet and most of them are confined to cramped, indoor living spaces called concentrated animal farming operations, or CAFOs.

Chickens are not supposed to be strictly vegetarians; their guts were meant for a more diverse diet. Chickens are omnivorous, meaning they eat a variety of plants, seeds, insects, and worms typically found in pastures. Sadly, the chickens of today are eating mostly corn, day in and day out.

Corn feed definitely provides ample calories, but *ample* is the operative word. The calorie-heavy and carb-rich corn causes the stationary chickens to bulk up quickly. Feeding chickens primarily corn produces an imbalance of omega-3 fats to omega-6 fats in their eggs. Healthy ratios should be between 1:2 and 1:4, but corn-fed chicken eggs have a ratio of up to 1:20. Omega-3 fats are important for cardiovascular health because they reduce inflammatory reactions, but too many omega-6 fats negate their benefit.

Conventionally raised chickens are stressed and tortured. Stop buying what comes out of them.

Thanks to the crowded conditions in the CAFOs, corn-fed chickens need regular doses of antibiotics and hormones in order to thwart the various infections that easily thrive in close quarters and to help increase their egg output.

In nature, wild hens only lay about 15 eggs per year. Thanks to decades of genetic manipulation, selective breeding, and hormone use, one hen can produce 250 to 300 eggs per year. This unnaturally high rate of egg-laying results in frequent disease and mortality.

Add to that the stress that these poor chickens undergo day in and day out thanks to the state of modern hen houses. About 95 percent of all egg-laying hens in this country—nearly 300 million birds—spend their lives in cages so small they can't even stretch their wings, and they share that tiny space with five to ten other birds. In these maddening conditions, hens will peck one another from stress, causing injury, infection and death.

Rather than give them more room, farmers cut off a portion of their sensitive beaks without painkiller. Many birds die of shock on the spot. When their production slows even little, they are stuffed conscious and headfirst into a "kill cone" to get their throats slit.

Now, you tell me that the output of these terrified, diseased chickens is something you should be putting into your body.

If you are not sensitive to eggs, please support farmers who let their hens roam free and eat plants, worm, and insects along with their organic feed. I know that organic, free range eggs can get expensive, so check out your local farmer's market and see if shopping locally can keep the cost down.

So, there you have it—all of the Sinister Seven and why they are problematic to you, your health, and your future. We mostly have modern farming practices to blame, and things are only getting worse each year.

Is there anything left to eat?

And how are you supposed to navigate this complex, toxic world?

A big part of your health begins with avoiding these seven foods. You do that, and you'll begin to heal. However, now let's fill in the gaps that these foods may leave in your life and talk about your Wild & Well game plan for making this new way of eating part of your lifestyle, not a fad.

SPECIAL BONUS SECTION

Eating Well in a Wild and Toxic World

It's such a complicated world that we live in.

As tempting as it may sound to some, there is no way to completely unplug and disengage from the rest of society forever. You may choose to live on a commune, grow your own food, and never have *any* interaction with the outside world in order to minimize your contact with

> **You can't obsess over every last decision you make all day long. You'll drive yourself crazy!**

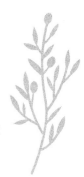

toxins and other environmental factors and influences—and if that describes you, then you are truly the epitome of the Wild & Well philosophy.

For the rest of us who have kids in school and jobs and a homeowner's association who won't allow us to raise goats and chickens in our backyards, what are we to do?

One answer is to recognize that you can't obsess over every last decision you make all day long. You'll drive yourself crazy!

We are all emotionally connected to food. We have meals on birthdays, at funerals and weddings, on Christmas and Thanksgiving, and on so many other occasions, from the significant to the everyday. Our entire world revolves around meals—and it should.

> **Your body likes *less*. It needs far *less* food than you give it, and it needs *less* fillers, fake ingredients, and taste enhancers.**

We are beautifully designed to break bread with people.

We are also supposed to enjoy life and not live each day obsessed with the macros of each meal. You know what that means? Have some chips and queso at the Super Bowl party, but then let that be your treat for the week. Enjoy a slice of gluten-free pumpkin pie with a little coconut whipped cream. Go to a cookout and eat a burger and have some potato chips. My goal is for you to have a resilient gut, so that when you do indulge in a meal that is not gluten, dairy, soy, corn, sugar, egg, and peanut free, you don't pay for it with your health the next week.

Then, the rest of the week, you know what you should be doing?

Cooking at home with as much organic, fresh, in season, one-ingredient foods as you can afford.

There's really nothing you can get outside of your own kitchen that will do you any favors. Restaurants want you to come back, so they make sure their food is really tasty. They do that with *more*—more fat, more salt, more sugar, more everything.

The problem is that your body likes *less*. It needs far *less* food than you give it, and it needs *less* fillers, fake ingredients, and taste enhancers.

While I'm not telling you to stop eating out, I will say that you should be making the lion's share of your meals at home.

I was listening to a podcast, and the creator of one of my favorite probiotics, Megaspore, was asked, "What is your health goal?"

He was silent for a few moments and then remarked with surprise that nobody's ever actually asked him about *his* gut goals. He responded by saying that he really just wants to be able to go to a restaurant and not be the guy who's calling the waiter aside to hear a breakdown of every ingredient in every dish. He wants to be the one who can go out with friends and order right off the menu—to have a burger and a bourbon with friends and have a gut that is resilient.

You don't have to live life in a bubble. You can go out and eat and belly laugh, and experience joy every single day! But if you want to live your life Wild & Well, it's time for a food makeover. It will require discipline, but if you are tired of being sick and tired, then today is the day you begin again. Here are a few simple steps to help you on this journey:

1. **Let go of perfection.** Before you can do *anything* else, you have to learn to cut yourself some slack. If you are prone to self-blame and being overly critical of your choices, you really need to let that crap go. Forgive yourself and resolve to be the kind of human being who loves life and goes out with friends from time to time. You will never be perfect because perfection is an illusion. There was only one perfect human—and it isn't you or me!

2. **Remove the Sinister Seven.** If you want to feel better, your critical step two is to focus on removal. Eliminate the Sinister Seven from your diet for at least three weeks. Eliminating the foods that cause an inflammatory response in your body is the biggest key to it all.

   You have to become a detective and figure out what is triggering inflammation in your body! Keep a detailed food diary to track your symptoms and when they occur. And remember, food sensitivities happen three hours to three days later (anywhere from three to seventy-two hours). So, if you have symptoms of joint pain today, it may be something you ate at breakfast or something you ate three days ago. Keep a detailed food diary to look back and identify the trigger.

3. **Do a detox.** Along with removal, I have all patients do a detox. In my practice, we use the Clear Change® 10-Day Program with UltraClear® RENEW from Metagenics. It's a ten-day metabolic detoxification program that leaves you feeling energized and helps decrease systemic inflammation so your body can begin to heal. I don't receive any money for recommending Metagenics, but feel free to do your own research on other detoxes on the market. Just make sure the ingredients are all clean, non-GMO.

Dani Recommends

The Ultra Clear Renew Detox is the best detox I have ever used, and I personally do it twice a year. **(DaniWilliamson.com/Wild)**

There is a big difference in a detox and a cleanse. A detox detoxifies the liver by taking fat-soluble toxins and making them water-soluble through a series of pathways. Cleanses generally rest the gut and are not detoxifying programs. You need a quality detox, not just a cleanse. I have a great FREE video on our Dani Williamson Wellness YouTube channel on our 10-day detox. There, you can watch and learn how a detoxification program is a huge kickstart to your healing. I detox first then transition to 21 days of eliminating the Sinister Seven foods for one solid month of decreasing inflammation.

4. **Stay the course.** Once the detox is over, you should continue refraining from the Sinister Seven for at least another three weeks—for a minimum of 31 total days of elimination of the top inflammatory foods. Your body is designed to heal itself, but you have to give it what it needs. This time of removal is the best way that I have found for patients to get a jumpstart on their restoration.

5. **Focus on single-ingredient foods.** During your 31-day removal and reset process, the focus will be on single-ingredient, lean, whole, real foods. God made food in the form it should be eaten—and it's as simple

as that. When you simplify and eat one-ingredient foods, that's when you begin to see changes.

During the reset and beyond, my rule of thumb on most food is this:

If it was made IN a plant and didn't come FROM a plant or FROM an animal, avoid it.

> **If it was made IN a plant and didn't come FROM a plant or FROM an animal, avoid it.**

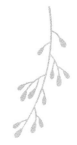

My own food style is like the Mediterranean diet. My primary meat of choice is wild-caught (never farm raised) fish. I also occasionally eat grass-fed beef and bison and free-range, organic chicken. I eat rice on occasion and consume plenty of heathy fats, fruits, and veggies.

Dani Recommends

Vital Choice is a phenomenal company that sells wild-caught fish such as salmon. **(DaniWilliamson.com for 5% discount)**

6. **Taste the rainbow.** The majority of my diet is a rainbow of colors. It contains lots of greens (and green juices), but also great blues and oranges and yellows and purples and reds. Add some variety and interest to your plate, and experiment with different veggies! I tell patients to add a new fruit or vegetable to their diet every time they visit the grocery store.

   I subscribe to Misfits Market weekly and get food I have never seen on a regular basis. It's fun Googling how to cook a ____. You can get 25 percent off your first order when you use the discount code COOKWME-IW4NDI at MisfitsMarket.com! The box is organic and contains ugly fruits and veggies that won't make to the store due to their appearance.

7. **Break out of ruts.** I read that most people feed their children the same five meals every day, year after year. This is not how we were meant to eat. Our bodies are designed for diversity, but we fall into bad habits and ruts.

   We eat the same few meals every week.

We wear the same three outfits in our closet.

We go to the same restaurants.

We vacation at the same places.

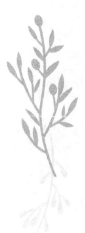

> **Plan your meals for the entire week. Make sure the list includes a rainbow of fresh produce. Stick to the list and also stick to the store's perimeter.**

I encourage you to break the cycle and try something new every week.

Routines and habits are good—until they aren't. Where do you instinctively gravitate to in the grocery store? If it's the middle aisles, the deli, the bakery, and the dairy section, those habits need to end. Here is your new game plan:

Plan your meals for the entire week. Make sure the list includes a rainbow of fresh produce. Stick to the list and also stick to the store's perimeter.

You may have to venture into the middle aisles for stuff like spices, olive oil, and trash bags, but the vast majority of your time should be spent on the perimeter edges of the store, where refrigeration is required and food lives that can easily spoil (meaning it's not stuffed with shelf stabilizers). Better yet, shop local and in season at your farmers market! If you don't have a local farmers market, then make sure you are buying in season. Strawberries are not designed to be eaten twelve months a year.

8. **Learn from Daniel.** Your diet will either heal you or kill you. That's the basis of The Daniel Plan in the Bible, too. If you aren't familiar with the story, here is the gist:

When Nebuchadnezzar became king in Jerusalem, he had his chief court official round up all the best and strongest men to serve in the palace. Among those chosen were Daniel and his friends, Shadrach, Meshach, and Abednego. All of the men were supposed to consume food and wine from the king's table, but Daniel did not want to defile his body with all of the rich foods, so he proposed a test to the chief official in Daniel 1:12-16:

> "Please test your servants for ten days: Give us nothing but vegetables to eat and water to drink. Then compare our appearance with that of the young men who eat the royal food and treat your servants in accordance with what you see."
>
> So, he agreed to this and tested them for ten days.
>
> At the end of the ten days they looked healthier and better nourished than any of the young men who ate the royal food. So the guard took away their choice food and the wine they were to drink and gave them vegetables instead.

After just *ten days* without the fatty foods and wine, meat, sugar, and dairy, Daniel and his friends looked noticeably better than the other strong and powerful servants!

That is the power of food—and that was 2,000 years ago. They weren't eating processed, packaged, bagged, canned, tubed, fake foods loaded with preservatives. Imagine how good he would feel now if he ate like that?

9. **Eat a Mediterranean Diet.** I have been eating a Mediterranean-style diet for years. It's a diet consisting of seasonal fruits and veggies, clean fats, nuts and seeds, wild caught fish, and a few gluten-free grains such as rice and quinoa.

Unfortunately, the FDA food pyramid recommendations have contradicted this style of eating for years. Their pyramid contains gluten and dairy, and it also recommends far too many grains and not enough healthy fats.

Needless to say, I have never supported the official food pyramid. So I decided to create my own to show the importance of a rainbow of veggies, clean protein, fresh fruit, and healthy fats. You'll find my superior version of the food pyramid on the next page (page 156).

At the bottom of my pyramid, I included the foundational pieces to a Wild & Well lifestyle: supplements, fats and oils, beverages, and my six steps. To download this Mediterranean nutrition prescription for free, visit DaniWilliamson.com/Wild.

DANI'S WILD & WELL

mediterranean
nutrition prescription

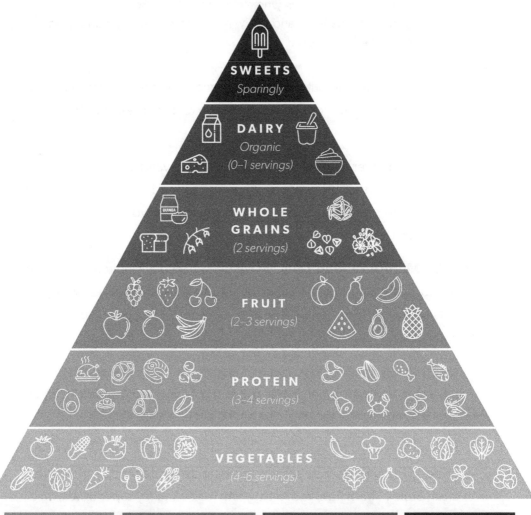

SWEETS
Sparingly

DAIRY
Organic
(0–1 servings)

WHOLE GRAINS
(2 servings)

FRUIT
(2–3 servings)

PROTEIN
(3–4 servings)

VEGETABLES
(4–6 servings)

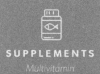

SUPPLEMENTS
Multivitamin
Vitamin D3
Omega 3s: EPA, DHA
Probiotic

HEALTHY FATS & OILS
Olive Oil (Extra-Virgin)
Grape Seed (Cold Pressed)
Ghee (Organic)

BEVERAGES
Water: 4–8 8oz. servings
Tea & Coffee: 0–3 servings
(<300mg Caffeine)
Alcohol: 0–2 servings

DANI'S SIX STEPS
Eat Well
Sleep Well
Move Well
Poop Well
DeStress Well
Commune Well

DANI'S TIPS FOR EATING WILD & WELL ON A BUDGET

I believe in all of my patients, and I believe in you. You already have everything you need to be well. You have a strong mind and a body that wants to regain balance and use its God-given systems to heal.

Eating well doesn't have to be hard, but it does take some re-education and, more importantly, some planning. If you have a family budget and do your best to stick to it every month, here are my tips for getting the most nutritional punch out of every dollar.

1. **Buy clean meat or don't eat meat.** If you can't afford to buy your meat, chicken, or fish grass-fed, pastured, or wild-caught, eat less of it and buy the best you can afford. Find a local farmer you trust that raises cattle, pork, and chickens and stock your freezer. Split a cow with a friend or family member. I don't eat a ton of red meat, but I do like a good steak on occasion.

2. **Cut your portions in half.** As a nation, we collectively eat far too much food. The next time you go to a restaurant, look around at the size of the meals that are being delivered to the tables. No one needs a salad that is 1,600 calories, so ask them to box half up of your meal BEFORE they bring it to the table. At home, use smaller plates. As the decades go by, our plates just keep getting bigger—just like our waist circumference.

THE HISTORY OF DINNER PLATE SIZE CORRESPONDS TO THE INCREASE IN OBESITY

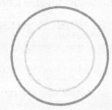

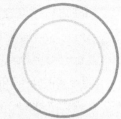

8.5 to 9-inch	**10-inch**	**11-inch**	**12-inch**
1960s. Holds about 800 cal.	*1980s. Holds about 1000 cal (20% increase).*	*2000s. Holds about 1600 cal (20% increase).*	*2009. Holds about 1900 cal (15% increase).*

3. **Shop and eat in season.** As you have probably noticed, produce prices fluctuate wildly throughout the year. Take some time to learn what's in season and what is being grown within 100 miles of you. For example, in many regions, Fall and Winter are ideal for root vegetables and nourishing soups and stews that include beets, parsnips, turnips, and carrots. Summertime is great for berries and melons.

Changing up your produce by season is a great way to keep your weekly menus diverse!

Good to Know

Go to TheSpruceEats.com for a seasonal produce guide that allows you to browse local foods by state!

4. **Spice it up.** I believe that herbs and spices are heavily underutilized in the U.S. I buy fresh turmeric at my local farmer's market and grate it to make broths loaded with garlic and ginger. All three of those ingredients (along with locally sourced, organic bone broth) are anti-inflammatory and loaded with antioxidants. Start using cinnamon, cayenne pepper, cloves, and sage. Rosemary is the only herb that my extremely non-green thumb can keep alive, and I have a rosemary bush as big as a couch at home.

5. **Drink clean water.** Many people know better than to drink tap water, but then those same people spend money every month buying plastic water bottles that clutter our landfills and oceans. Tap water is not a solution, but neither are bottles. Berkey makes a great water filter and includes an optional fluoride filter. There are also affordable under-the-sink options for reverse osmosis systems. Last year, the office staff at Integrative Family Medicine gave me a Puremaster V Series whole-house filter with additional fluoride filter for my house. It filters out pharmaceuticals, fluoride, chlorine, chloride, heavy metals, pesticides, and more! I now drink, cook, shower, and bathe with clean water. What an amazing gift that was—the gift of health.

> ### *Dani Recommends*
> Fiji is my go-to water brand when I'm out and about and need to hydrate. For everyday use, I like the Hydro Flask reusable water bottles made from stainless steel or just a large glass mason jar.

Plastic water bottles are really not a good solution over the long haul. If you do need to drink from a plastic bottle, make sure that the bottle does not contain bisphenol A or BPA, which is an endocrine disruptor that creates inflammation in the body.

Buying a water filtration system is an investment up front, but, over time, you will save money and the planet. Since you should be drinking half of your body weight in ounces every day, you need a long-term solution for clean water. The reason I got a whole-house water filtration system was the light bulb moment I had when I realized I filtered my drinking water but bathed and showered under contaminated water daily.

6. **Shop around.** I started shopping at Aldi when I was on food stamps and continue to shop there today. They have a large organic selection that seems to be growing by the week! If you didn't know, Aldi actually owns Trader Joe's, which is known for its quality food and great prices.

Even on a tight budget, you can feed your family well. My kids and I were on food stamps and used a medical card for five years, and the entire time, I had no idea I could have been using my food stamps at many farmers' markets.

There are solutions for every budget, if you are willing to invest a little time and energy into finding the best options near you.

SEEING IS BELIEVING

The literature and research are strong on the inflammatory effects of the Sinister Seven—but here's some real talk: While taking a deeper dive into the research on each food, I discovered that, honestly, you can find studies to support any theory you have. The good. The bad.

Soy is good for you. Soy will make our sons grow breasts.

Dairy is perfectly healthy. Dairy will be the death of us all.

Corn feed does not change the nutritional value of eggs. Corn feed is causing the chickens and us to all get fat and diseased.

I can't do much about study biases, false reporting, and crooked motives. What I can do is tell you what the removal of the Sinister Seven has done for me and thousands of my patients. I see people who are healing every day!

> **Change your diet and you change the entire trajectory of your and your family's lives and possibly future generations— and to me, that's exciting.**

If you want to justify your desire for cheese and aren't willing to give it up, there is no doubt that you can find a study to support that. Studies are fraught with biases—and always look at the fine print on precisely *who* funded the study.

What doesn't ever lie is how YOU feel.

Don't blindly trust me or any study in this book. See for yourself. Remove the Sinister Seven for 21 days and see how you feel. I wager it will be the best you've felt in decades.

Still, don't expect miracles. It took your body years to get into this state, so it will understandably take some time to get out.

Experts predict that today's children will be the first generation that are going to die before their parents in the U.S.

That's not acceptable.

We are destroying the health of our kids by feeding them packaged, processed, bagged, canned, tubed, fake food. They are not eating things that bring health to the body. They're not even eating anything that looks like food.

Change your diet and you change the entire trajectory of your and your family's lives and possibly future generations—and to me, that's exciting.

It all starts with you and your desire to be Wild & Well.

wild & well Rx

Dani Williamson, MSN, FNP

R**x** Patient Name: ....

Age: ....   Date: ....

1. Read this chapter again before you go forward. If you don't think the food industry is controlling your health, you are mistaken.

2. Look at every ingredient on your package if you aren't ready to give up processed foods. Then consider whether you want to put those ingredients in your body or your child's body.

3. Keep a food diary for 21 days. Food sensitivities are delayed three hours to three days later. If you have a headache today, it could be something you ate days ago.

4. Find your local farmer's market and get to know your farmers.

5. Make a commitment to only eat in season and foods grown as close to home as possible (preferably less than 100 miles).

6. Cut out just one food at a time if the thought of cutting out the top seven inflammatory foods overwhelms you.

7. Bring healthier food choices into your home as you run out of processed, fake, bagged, canned, man-made food.

8. Get the kids involved in food shopping and cooking. It will change their lives!

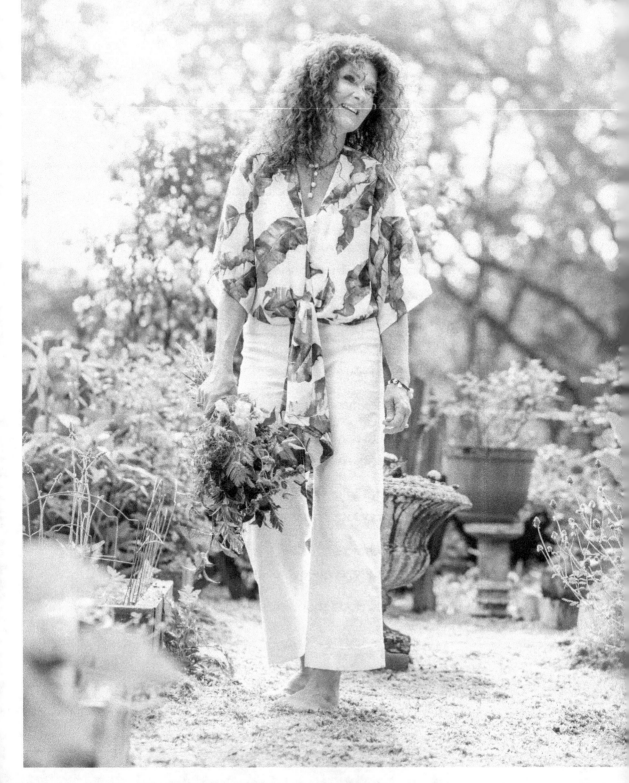

"Create a sanctuary in your bedroom that is meant for sleep and sex only."

CHAPTER 6

sleep well

"I love sleep. My life has the tendency to
fall apart when I'm awake, you know?"
ERNEST HEMINGWAY

Thomas Alva Edison is considered by some to be the greatest inventor of all time. During his remarkable life and career, he received an astonishing 1,093 patents. Edison developed a method for recording sound. He is responsible for coming up with the technology that helped bring the light bulb to the masses. He was the first person to project a motion picture.

I don't think there is a human being alive who would dispute the importance that Edison played in America's technological revolution. He helped set the stage for the modern electric world in which we live today!

Edison was also once quoted as saying, "Sleep is a criminal waste of time, inherited from our cave days."

Oh, well. I guess even the brightest minds among us can get it wrong from time to time.

No disrespect to Edison, but this is a dangerous mistruth, one that is contradicted by massive amounts of science, studies, and evidence. In many ways, it is the light bulb (and electricity itself) that is responsible for negatively altering the way we, as a species, sleep.

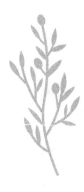

Think about this: Before we lit up our homes, humans based their patterns on the rising and setting of the sun.

Think about this: Before we lit up our homes, humans based their patterns on the rising and setting of the sun.

Families were up at sunrise and then went to bed not long after it went back down. With no TVs or smartphones to distract them, there wasn't a whole lot to do after the daylight was gone.

Sleep was once highly revered by all. From the beginning of recorded time, sleep and dreams have played essential roles in virtually every culture and religion. The ancient Egyptians worshipped Euf Ra, the god of sleep, rest, peace, and courage. They saw sleep as a healing tool, and they used it as a method of healing in special *sleep temples*, designed for a modality they called "dream incubation."

In Greek mythology, Hypnos was the god of sleep. His mother was Nyx (night), and his father was Erebus (darkness). Even Zeus, king of the gods, was afraid of Nyx because the night is so powerful. Hypnos himself was said to own half of every human life because of the tremendous role that sleep plays in life span.

In the Bible, God loved using nighttime and the dream state to reveal essential messages to important people. He spoke via dreams to Jacob, Joseph, and Pharaoh in Genesis; to Solomon and Daniel; and to Joseph and the Wise Men about Jesus' birth.

In order to do a good day's work, our ancestors knew they needed a good night's sleep.

Ironically, it is because of modern society's tireless pursuit of success that getting sleep has now taken a backseat to burning the midnight oil. As you may be able to guess, the idiom "burning the midnight oil" comes from the fact that candles and oil lamps were once the only forms of light after dark. English author Francis Quarles first used the phrase in 1635 to refer to working late by candlelight—an act that used to have a formal name, which was to "elucubrate."

That's a ten-dollar word for a gal from Gilbertsville, Kentucky!

Today, we "elucubrate" every night, but by the light of our laptops, computers, phones, TVs, lamps, light fixtures, streetlights, city lights, alarm clocks, stoves, noise machines, diffusers, salt lamps, and every other electronic gadget in our house with a "power on" light.

> In order to do a good day's work, our ancestors knew they needed a good night's sleep.

We feel this incredible pressure to stay up late and get stuff done. This pressure is exacerbated by images of relentless millionaire entrepreneurs who "rise and grind" and parents who *appear* to keep a spotless house, put their superstar kids in three sports a piece, and also manage to have a date night every week.

You may be interested in finding out that before artificial lighting, entire cultures engaged in something called *segmented sleep*. That is, they went to bed at dusk, awakened four or so hours later to relax, have sex, or do a chore by candlelight, and then fell back asleep for another four hours until sunrise.

There are also numerous accounts from medical texts and court records across cultures that reference a "first" and "second" sleep.

Historian A. Roger Ekirch's book, *At Day's Close: Night in Times Past*, describes how entire households once retired a couple of hours after dusk, woke a few hours later for one to two hours, and then had a second sleep until dawn.

Ekirch found that references to the first and second sleep started to disappear during the late 17th century and were almost entirely gone by the 19th century.

What's the most fascinating about this to me is that the increased appearance of "insomnia" in literature in the late 19th century just so happens to coincide with the period where accounts of split sleep disappeared. It's as though society started placing unnecessary pressure on individuals to achieve continuous, consolidated sleep every night—which added to the anxiety about sleep and perpetuated the problem.

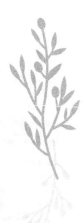

> **When I learned about first and second sleep, I began to realize that how you sleep may not be nearly as important as how you feel when you wake up.**

I am guilty of telling my patients in the past that the only way to sleep is to get a solid eight hours of uninterrupted shuteye a night.

When I learned about first and second sleep, I began to realize that how you sleep may not be nearly as important as how you feel when you wake up.

In other words, do you awaken rested, refreshed, and ready for the day?

I'm *not* saying that from now on, you should go to bed at dusk, wake up at midnight to have sex, and then go to sleep again until dawn (unless, of course, that sounds fun to you). What I *am* saying is that it's not merely the pressure of working hard or having too many responsibilities that is keeping us awake.

We are also stressed out by the increased pressure to sleep! And, truly, I'm sorry to every one of you that I pressured to sleep all night long.

By now, thanks to the prevalence of reports and articles on the subject, it should be no surprise that every expert agrees on one thing: you need seven to eight hours of sleep a night (maybe not in a row, but that is the total) for optimal health and function.

Particularly over the past decade, we've seen a tidal wave of new research, all showing the multifaceted importance of sleep to human performance. So much so that the famous adage "I'll sleep when I'm dead" has become "I'll (quite literally) sleep my way to the top."

Without proper sleep, your body will never thrive, and it will certainly never heal. Far from simply being something you do in order not to "feel tired," sleep is the ultimate wellness cure. When you get enough of it at the right time, it's the most potent human performance enhancer in the world.

If this is the case—and we all know it is—then what in the world is our problem? Why are zzzs so hard to come by for so many? It's a complicated answer, so just keep reading.

The Sad State of Modern Sleep

There are more than 2,800 sleep clinics in the U.S. that generated an estimated $7.1 billion in revenue in 2015. Sleep clinics are continuing to grow by around 4 percent every year for the last five years, and this growth is expected to continue.

We now have highly paid sleep gurus, corporate classes, and even sleep retreats. Whole holidays exist for you to be unconscious as much as possible. We can track our sleep via apps and mats and rings that rank and rate our sleep. We can enhance it by white noise and pink noise and brown noise and green noise and possibly some other colors, too.

Mattress companies were suddenly tech start-ups. There are high-tech pillows and mood-altering blankets and "smart" pajamas endorsed by pro-football stars. One mattress even scolds you for not lying on it enough. There are bestselling sleep books and a sleep podcast—Sleep With Me (downloaded around two million times a month) that hopes you miss how it ends, since the obvious goal is to be sleeping by then.

It is an industry estimated to be worth more than $120 billion.

Sleep is big business—and for a reason.

According to the most recent studies, an estimated 28 to 44 percent of the population experience a shortened sleep duration, which is considered to be less than seven hours.[212]

Almost half of our population (48 percent) report nightly snoring. Additionally, a staggering 37.9 percent of Americans have unintentionally fallen asleep during the day at least one time in the preceding month. In fact, I have a patient who got fired because she fell asleep at her computer while at work. My own mother has always fallen asleep sitting up. She fell asleep in middle of physical therapy more than once at her assisted living home!

This is a problem—and it's not just affecting our moods or our ability to do our jobs.

First, there's the weight gain. In the past six years, researchers had found that cravings for junk food increase 45 percent for the under slept. Lack of sleep swells the hormone for appetite and, worse, limits the hormone for satisfaction, so we don't feel full even after eating. The result: We don't know when to stop.

Next, you have increased dementia risk. In the past seven years, scientists have determined that cerebrospinal fluids were pushed up during the night in order to wash out all the toxins the brain created by thinking during the day. The degradation of this process—a process that naturally happens with age but is exacerbated by simply sleeping less—dramatically increases the risk of dementia and Alzheimer's.

I wonder if part of my mother's dementia is related to the fact that she has never been a good sleeper. All my life, I remember her staying up until the wee hours of the morning watching old movies and TV.

Third, you have overall diminished mental and physical health. Research found that your stresses through the day are replayed during REM sleep at night (as dreams), but with the stress hormones switched off. So, it allows you to take perspective and reset yourself emotionally. When you don't get enough sleep, those stressors stay front and center in your conscious mind.

Put simply: The less you sleep, the less you live.

What about overall health and wellness? Routinely sleeping less than six or seven hours annihilates your immune system. It doubles your risk of cancer and increases the likelihood of your coronary arteries becoming brittle and blocked, leading to cardiovascular disease, strokes, and congestive heart failure.

Put simply: The less you sleep, the less you live.

Unfortunately, devotees of the "I'll sleep when I'm dead" ideology will likely get their wish sooner rather than later. Diet and exercise are commonly thought to have the biggest impact on health, but the reality is it's not even close. If you're missing sleep to get up for the gym, you'd be better off staying in bed.

Tiredness is the new norm. On any given day, ask a group of friends how they are feeling, and a notable number of them will reply with *exhausted, tired, stressed, worn down, sleep-deprived*, or some variety.

In my office, well over half of my patients tell me they don't feel they get enough sleep. The primary reasons are going to bed too late and suffering from insomnia due to either a known reason (such as a medical condition or anxiety) or an unknown reason. Perhaps more disturbing is that even fewer of my patients say they wake up feeling refreshed in the morning.

The Shocking Truth About Daylight Saving Time

- In the Spring, when most people lose an hour of sleep due to daylight saving, the rate of heart attacks increases by 25 percent!

- The minimal sleep loss associated with the spring shift to Daylight Saving Time produces a short-term increase of the likelihood of accidental vehicular death, while the fall shift has little effect on vehicle-related fatalities.

- Data suggests that increased sleep fragmentation and sleep latency present a cumulative effect of sleep loss, at least across the following week, perhaps longer.

- The autumn transition is often popularized as a gain of one hour of sleep, but there is little evidence of extra sleep on that night.

Sources cited for above: [213,214,215]

The Age of Sleep Disorders

Unlike anatomy, sleep is a relatively new science. In fact, it was only about a hundred years ago that Dr. Nathaniel Kleitman, known as "the father of American sleep research," began questioning the inner workings of sleep and circadian rhythms. The landmark discovery of rapid eye movement (REM) during sleep wasn't made until 1953 by Dr. Kleitman and one of his students, Dr. Eugene Aserinsky.

Another of Dr. Kleitman's students, Dr. William C. Dement, extended Kleitman's research. Dement described the "cyclical" nature of nocturnal sleep in 1955 and established the relationship between REM sleep and dreaming in 1958. At that point, Dement published a paper on the existence of a cyclic organization of sleep in cats. This finding (that animals other than humans have sleep cycles) created an explosion of fundamental research that united researchers from many different fields including electro-physiology, pharmacology, biochemistry, and chronobiology (aka circadian rhythms).

This new science, known as *sleep medicine*, has rapidly evolved over the past twenty-five or so years based on the convergence of major developments and discoveries about all that happens when we sleep. It's a "new" science that is devoted to learning more about something that has been happening to humans since Adam and Eve.

Today, sleep research comprises many different areas: narcolepsy research; sleep and cardio-respiratory research; and studies of pain and sleep, circadian rhythms, shift work and its effects on sleep, sleep deprivation, sleep and aging, and infant sleep, to name a few. There are more than two hundred accredited sleep disorders centers and laboratories in the U.S. alone, all designed to recognize and treat sleep disorders.

While the discoveries about the mechanisms of sleep may be more recent, what is not new is the understanding that sleep is important and that anything standing in its way is harmful. And that leads us into the issue of sleep disorders.

Sleep disorders are not new, nor rare. They are pervasive! The three most common sleep disorders are:

1. INSOMNIA
Insomnia is the most common sleep disorder. It is best characterized as the inability to fall asleep or stay asleep, or waking too early in the morning. Now, I want you to understand something very important: Insomnia is almost *always* a symptom rather than an isolated diagnosis.

Chronic sleep disruptions such an insomnia are often indicators of underlying medical or psychological problems, such as other more serious sleep disorders, depression, and anxiety.[216] Insomnia could also be a side effect of thyroid issues, fluctuations in sex hormones, and much more.

Depression and insomnia are inextricably linked. A large retrospective study (including 15,000 subjects) in four European countries found that *chronic insomnia* (defined as insomnia lasting more than six months) appeared before the onset of depression/mood disorder in 41.7 percent of cases. Similar numbers were noted for anxiety disorder.[217]

Other studies suggest that insomnia suffers are 10 times more likely to suffer from clinical depression and 17 times more likely to have clinical anxiety.[218]

Insomnia is also a significant cause of morbidity and mortality. The direct and indirect costs of insomnia place a tremendous economic burden on society and employers. In addition to the cost of medical treatments and drugs, measurable costs of insomnia include reduced productivity and increased absenteeism, accidents, and hospitalizations. Insomnia also results in additional medical costs due to increased morbidity and mortality, depression due to insomnia, and increased alcohol consumption.[219]

If that's not enough to scare you to sleep, I'm not sure what is.

But that's kind of the point, isn't it? We all know that sleep is important. In fact, the pressure to sleep is often so great that it keeps us awake. How's that for irony?

I will discuss my "remedies" for insomnia at the end of this chapter, so stay tuned.

2. SLEEP APNEA

Obstructive sleep apnea (OSA) is a disorder that stems from disruption to the respiratory system during sleep and causes intermittent airflow blockage throughout the night, with or without you ever even being aware of it. OSA is the most common form of sleep apnea and is estimated to affect approximately 4 percent of men and 2 percent of women (or one out of about every twelve people).

There is another less common type of apnea called central sleep apnea. It is also a disorder in which your breathing repeatedly stops and starts during sleep. With OSA, breathing stops and starts because the airway is narrowed or blocked. However, central sleep apnea occurs because your brain doesn't send proper signals to the muscles that control your breathing. This type of apnea is seen in patients with brain stem injuries, those who are severely obese, and sometimes in patients who abuse narcotic painkillers.

OSA has been associated with age, obesity, structural issues, alcohol use, drug use, and smoking. It's important to note that just because you snore, it does not automatically mean you suffer from sleep apnea.

My next-door neighbor suddenly and tragically lost her husband at age 27 to obstructive sleep apnea. He was the love of her life, and his death was unnecessary and possibly could have been prevented. He refused to go for surgery that was needed to improve his OSA. He used his CPAP nightly and did the night he died, but he would take it off in the night.

It is believed that only about 10 percent of people with OSA seek treatment, leaving the majority of OSA sufferers undiagnosed. Considering experts say that untreated sleep apnea can rob you of years of your life, that sounds pretty dangerous and irresponsible. Here's how they explained it:

> "The DNA in the cells of those who left their sleep apnea untreated was 'aging' faster than it should. As DNA ages, cells begin to break down, and health risk for cancer and chronic disease goes up. Many of these diseases, including the untreated sleep apnea, have the potential to shorten your lifespan."[220]

Another reason for OSA being linked to decreased lifespan is the fact that it causes low grade chronic inflammation. This is not surprising, considering it may contribute to the development of multiple sclerosis (MS) and diabetes.[221] And, people with OSA are 10 times more likely to suffer from depression.[222] Studies also show that long-time sufferers of OSA are also more likely to have cardiovascular disease.[223] The common signs of sleep apnea are:[224]

- Waking up with a very sore or dry throat.

- Loud snoring.

- Occasionally waking up with a choking or gasping sensation.

- Sleepiness or lack of energy during the day.

- Sleepiness while driving.

- Morning headaches.

- Restless sleep.

- Forgetfulness, mood changes, and a decreased interest in sex.

If you have even a few of these symptoms, I recommend getting tested at an inpatient sleep lab. If you go through the proper channels and an ENT recommends this course of action, most insurance plans will cover your examination.

It's too important to ignore. Talk to someone about this before it robs you of years of your life.

3. RESTLESS LEGS SYNDROME

Another disorder that is keeping you from getting the sleep you need is restless legs syndrome. Restless leg syndrome (RLS) is characterized by a typically insurmountable urge to shake or move the legs. RLS affects many people outside the realm of sleep issues, but a portion of those suffering tend to see flare-ups mostly during long periods of stillness, especially sleep.

The true causes of RLS are not widely known or accepted, but health experts believe that irregular hyperexcitability along the spinal cord may lead to sporadic arm and leg movements.

One possible cause of RLS is an iron deficiency or iron absorption problems that may lead to the onset of both restless legs and even restless arms. Other triggering factors could include:[225]

- Sleep deprivation

- Iron deficiency/anemia

- Chronic alcoholic consumption

- Renal failure

- Parkinson's disease

- Diabetes

- Peripheral nerve disorder

- The use of certain medications such as antidepressants, antipsychotic medications, anti-allergic medications, etc.

- Pregnancy, especially during the last trimester of pregnancy

Just like insomnia and sleep apnea, people with RLS often feel its effects during the day in the form of tiredness, grumpiness, and difficulty concentrating. Most look to treat moderate RLS with home practices such as stretching, massage, and ice or heat packs, but extreme cases may require specialized medical care.

The Sleep Aid Trap

It is probably not surprising to discover that sleep disorders and mental health disorders are linked. Recent research is still attempting to determine (in true "chicken or the egg" fashion) whether disrupted sleep is a symptom of mental health issues, or whether mental health issues are the consequences of chronic disordered sleep.

> **A drug-based approach to sleep issues is only making things worse for bedtime and beyond.**

There are a number of studies that link insomnia with an increased risk of dementia, but what about the other way around?[226,227] More and more research is now confirming what many have suspected for some time— that habitual users of drugs such as Ambien and even Benadryl for insomnia have a significantly increased risk of developing dementia and Alzheimer's.

A landmark study first released at the Alzheimer's Association International Conference 2019 reported that older adults who habitually use some type of sleep medication were 43 percent more likely to develop dementia than those who took them "rarely" or never. This is particularly true among older white adults. The reason this is truer for white people is currently unclear.[228]

But isn't it a simple solution to a major problem? We need sleep! So, why not take a pill and get some much-needed rest and repair?

It's tempting. I know. I've done it.

The problem is that, over time, chemical sleep aids simply do not work or, perhaps more accurately, may cause more problems than they solve.

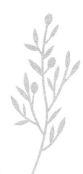

There is no way to sugarcoat it. Sleep aids don't provide enough benefits to outweigh their many downsides.

A drug-based approach to sleep issues is only making things worse for bedtime and beyond.

Additionally, as of 2019, there are now black box warnings on several of the most common sleep drugs, including eszopiclone (Lunesta), zaleplon (Sonata), and zolpidem (Ambien, Ambien CR, Edluar, Intermezzo, and Zolpimist). The warnings were added because of an alarming number of patients who took one of these hypnotics and displayed "complex sleep behaviors" that included turning on ovens, driving cars, and shooting themselves with guns.[229]

One of my most concerning issues with prescription drugs for insomnia as well as for depression and is that these drugs suppress rapid eye movement (REM) sleep, which is a process that is vitally important for brain function. In fact, two types of sleep aids—selective serotonin reuptake inhibitors (SSRIs) and tricyclic antidepressants (TCA)—were shown to inhibit REM sleep by 84 and 69 percent respectively.[230]

So, you take a drug such as Ambien thinking it's going to help you get some shut eye, but then you really don't sleep all that much better *and* you suppress your deep REM sleep—which is the time when your body actually heals and makes oxytocin, and your hormones start to reset and get ready for the next day.[231]

There is no way to sugarcoat it. Sleep aids don't provide enough benefits to outweigh their many downsides.

When I was going through my divorce, I took Ambien for a few weeks. It was supposed to help me sleep better. Did it help? A little, I guess. To me, the difference was barely noticeable and not worth the risks and side effects and a potential dependency.

If you frequently travel overseas, prescription sleep aids may be your lifeline thanks to the regular jump in time zones. If you are currently using sleep aids, please understand that this is not a reprimand of occasional use—the problem is that the research just doesn't pan out for long-term use and actually serves in many cases to make the problem worse.

You weren't born with insomnia or restless legs. You also most likely were not born with sleep apnea. Something or some things turned on these issues in your body.

So, what is the root cause? Why are you not sleeping?

There could be so many reasons! Of course, figuring it out is like trying to solve a Rubik's cube and get all of those colors aligned perfectly.

I get it, because I've been there, too.

Is it hormonal? A lot of women sleep better with more progesterone. Is it stress related? Life in these modern times is certainly no cake walk. Is it your adrenals? We're all running crazy and exhausted!

Do you have a deficiency that is causing you to be unable to rest well? I recommend checking your magnesium RBC, vitamin D3, and iron levels. One of the biggest culprits behind restless legs is anemia caused by an iron deficiency. Another way to help is by taking magnesium RBC, which is a smooth muscle relaxer (that's also why it helps you poop).

These are all issues worth pursuing, and I highly recommend speaking with a functional medicine provider about getting tested in each of these areas and more. So, with that in mind, we are going to spend the next few sections discussing two of the greatest saboteurs of sleep: your adrenals and your hormones.

Hormones and Sleep

Your sleep-wake cycle follows what is known as a "circadian rhythm," which is probably a term you've heard before. Put simply, your circadian rhythm dictates your body's 24-hour sleep-wake cycle, and here's what's interesting:

Your body's cortisol production follows a similar circadian rhythm.

Why does this matter? To understand that, you have to know that *cortisol* is a hormone that is produced by a complex network known as the hypothalamic pituitary adrenal (HPA) axis.

CORTISOL: THE STRESS HORMONE

The HPA axis includes your hypothalamus and pituitary gland, both of which are in your brain—and it also includes your adrenal glands. They are the glands that produce the hormone cortisol (aka the stress hormone) through a complex series of body signals.

Maintaining proper cortisol production is important because sleep and the stress response share the same pathway: that HPA axis I mentioned above. When something disrupts the HPA axis functions, it disrupts your sleep cycles as well.

Cortisol production drops to its lowest point around midnight, and then it maxes out about an hour after waking. For many of us, that peak is around 9:00 a.m. In addition to the circadian cycle, around fifteen to eighteen smaller pulses of cortisol are released throughout the day and night. Some of those smaller bursts of cortisol correspond to shifts in your sleep cycles.

It would be so easy to understand it all if it were as simple as "the body goes to sleep, repairs and resets, and then you wake up bright eyed and bushy tailed."

However, it's not that simple, because sleep is not a steady state of rest. Your body goes through various stages of sleep every night. A sleep cycle lasts about an hour and a half, and during each cycle, you experience three stages of non-REM (non-rapid eye movement) sleep followed by REM (rapid eye movement) sleep, which is the part of your sleep cycle where you have vivid dreams.

We have disrupted this cycle in our modern lives with various things: computers, lights, TVs, electromagnetic fields (EMFs), etc. Studies have shown that insomnia and other forms of sleep deprivation cause your body to secrete more cortisol during the day, perhaps in an effort to stimulate alertness.

The problem is that disrupted cortisol levels don't only impact your ability to sleep. Unfortunately, they can also affect other aspects of your health. For instance, disrupted cortisol levels can cause:

* Metabolic disorders.

* Weight gain.

* Inflammation.

* Cognitive decline.

* Anxiety and depression.

* Headaches.

* Heart disease.

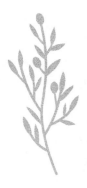

Your body does not know the difference between good and bad stress.

There are a lot of things you can do to positively affect your cortisol levels, but the biggest two are eating well and effectively managing your stress load.

Stress causes a spike in cortisol, and here's something I didn't even learn until AFTER nursing school: Your adrenals shoot out cortisol when you're under any stress at all, good or bad. Here is what's crazy:

Your body does not know the difference between good and bad stress.

The body doesn't know that you're getting married. That's a great stressor, but still technically stress. Conversely, it also doesn't know that your fiancé just got into a car accident. The body can't discern that stress from any other form. It just looks at both instances as "stress."

So, the way you *manage* all forms of stress—the good and the bad—is key, as it will disrupt your sleep tremendously if your cortisol levels are dysfunctional for any reason.

There's a great book called *Why Zebras Don't Get Ulcers*, from which I learned that when zebras run from a lion or other predator, their cortisol level shoots through the roof. Then, when the threat's over, they go right back to normal. Humans don't operate that way, do we?

We feel stressed in the morning as we think about all we have to do that day.

We stress about making it to work on time or getting the kids to school.

We stress when there's a wreck on the interstate.

We stress when the fridge breaks.

We stress when the kids get sick.

We stress when we are planning for a birthday party.

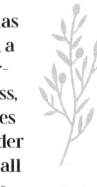

Modern life has most of us in a state of near-constant stress, and our bodies are failing under the weight of all that pressure.

We stress as we lay in bed at night thinking about what did or didn't happen that day or what's on the agenda for the next day.

Modern life has most of us in a state of near-constant stress, and our bodies are failing under the weight of all that pressure.

I am a big believer in testing, not guessing, your adrenals and cortisol levels. So, get tested and see what you're dealing with! Balancing your cortisol levels can take time, but, while you're working on it, good sleep hygiene (which you'll learn all about in a few minutes) can work wonders.

OXYTOCIN: THE LOVE HORMONE

Another hormone I want to highlight is oxytocin, otherwise known as the love hormone. Your body produces it when you get a good night's sleep, when you have sex, when you snuggle on the couch, when you hug someone, or when you nurse a child, among other actions.

Levels of oxytocin peak around five hours after going to sleep. That is during the REM sleep cycle, as a rule. It's also when sex dreams happen. Interestingly, orgasms and erections in the night are associated with the release of oxytocin during the REM cycle.

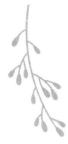

We clearly need more oxytocin in our lives! Translation: We need more sex.

Oxytocin is becoming more and more understood just in the last few decades. Research shows that oxytocin can help reduce stress. A 2007 study reported that after prairie voles (who are monogamous) exhibited signs of anxiety, stress, and depression from being separated from their partners, they were injected with oxytocin and experienced reduced symptoms and an overall calmer demeanor.[232]

Oxytocin also induces sleep. Oxytocin released in the brain under stress-free conditions naturally promotes sleep, according to a 2003 animal study.[233] This just makes sense, considering the fact that we now know that oxytocin counters the effects of cortisol, the stress hormone.

Experts have even been able to show in animal studies that increased levels of oxytocin during sleep help reduce obstructive sleep apnea (OSA).[234]

We clearly need more oxytocin in our lives! Translation: We need more sex.

I know some of my married female readers just rolled their eyes, but just hear me out. Ladies, your husband wants more sex (this is not a surprise, I'm guessing). And you should want more sex, too! Not only does it solidify your bond, but it also keeps you healthier and helps you both sleep like logs.

You may be in a phase of life where you just aren't "feeling it." Stress and babies and hormones and a full calendar can do that. That is when you need to start getting creative. Do the work to make sex *fun* again. I know, it's a contradiction... do "work" to make sex fun.

But anything truly great in life requires some work! This applies to many things including your relationships, your career, your kids, your health, and your sex life.

There are usually two ways to a man's heart: Feed him well and keep him happy in bed. Good sex starts in the kitchen before everyone leaves for work in the morning. Set your morning up to have a good evening. Smack his butt or give him a passionate kiss, not just a peck (something that lets him know what's waiting for him later that night).

Start texting your husband while he's at work and see how happy he is to come home that evening and know what kind of night he's going to have. Be willing to be naked and not in total darkness so he can see you. I promise he'll love what he sees.

This is not some altruistic thing you are "doing" for your guy. It's great for you, too! You'll both sleep better and feel a level of intimacy in your marriage that all the forces on earth couldn't break apart.

All of my married patients love to tell me, "Oh, Dani, just wait until you're married again. You'll be singing a different tune."

Well, I've been married, and I've also experienced what the lack of sex does to a marriage. I won't ever let that happen again. Sex certainly can't *make* a marriage, but the lack of it will absolutely *break* it apart.

If you're married to a good man who loves you for you, return the favor and give him what he needs to feel loved (sex is almost every man's love language… not all, but most).

I know this isn't the most scientific topic, but it needed to be said. I hope you'll hear me and start making your man feel wanted and desired again!

ESTROGEN: THE DEVIL HORMONE

Okay, I'm kidding about the title. However, ask any woman over the age of 35 how she feels about estrogen, and you'll get responses that range from maniacal laughter to crying or maybe even a little screaming.

Y'all, estrogen can make us ladies crazy! The unfortunate thing is it's also a major contributor to sleep issues among middle-aged and older females. Here are a few stats to let you know what we're dealing with:

Perimenopause

- 56 percent of perimenopausal women sleep less than seven hours on average (versus pre-menopausal women at 33 percent)

- 24.8 percent report trouble falling asleep

- 30.8 percent have trouble staying asleep

- 50 percent wake up feeling tired (versus rested) four or more days/week

Menopause

- 40.5 percent of postmenopausal women sleep less than seven hours on average

- 27.1 percent report difficulty falling asleep

- 35.9 percent difficulty staying asleep

- 55 percent wake tired

That's a lot of women waking up tired after a rough night of sleep.

Now, although I jokingly called estrogen the "devil hormone," I want to make sure we don't jump on the train of demonizing estrogen. Estrogen is good for sleep, mood, and libido. Our main estrogen—estradiol—sensitizes the brain to oxytocin and dopamine and also triggers the release of serotonin.

It supports healthy mood and sleep and is also important for skin, bone health, insulin sensitivity, and metabolic rate. Too little can cause depression and severe insomnia, which is why taking estrogen can relieve those symptoms. Conversely, when estrogen is too high (especially compared to progesterone), it can cause symptoms such as headaches, insomnia, and more.

Still, it always seems like we've got too much estrogen or not enough. Lower levels of estrogen have been shown to contribute to moderate to severe obstructive sleep apnea (OSA) in perimenopausal and menopausal women.[235] And higher levels of estrogen can cause sleeping problems—either an increased need for sleeping and fatigue or insomnia, because it stimulates the nervous system. A person with high estrogen experiences mood swings, and increased stress levels delay sleep onset.[236]

Estrogen is a hormone that you would be wise to keep in check. That is why I always say get tested! **Don't just start a progesterone cream because your friend did, and she lost weight.** Do it right and get tested. We'll talk more about progesterone in the supplements section toward the end of the chapter.

The Early Risers Club

It's not just women who have more sleep issues as they age. A 2005 National Sleep Foundation poll found that 38 percent of all people older than 54 were more likely to say they wake up frequently during the night, versus 24 percent of 18 to 29-year-olds, 31 percent of 30 to 49-year-olds, and 33 percent of 50 to 54-year-olds. [237,238]

Something else happens as we age that you may or may not have started to notice. As we grow older, most of us start going to bed earlier and also getting up earlier. Why does this happen? No one knows for sure. However, I do know one thing that is certain:

> No matter our age, we'd all benefit greatly from this type of "early to bed, early to rise" sleep schedule.

No matter our age, we'd all benefit greatly from this type of "early to bed, early to rise" sleep schedule.

A recent study showed that students who get up earlier have higher GPAs.[239] Kids that are lifelong members of the elite "Early Risers Club" feel better and perform better. The same study also reported that morning people anticipate problems better and handle work crises better as well.

Early birds are apparently more proactive than evening people, and they tend to do well in business.

I'm a lifelong member of the Early Risers club, and so are my kids. Maybe it's just the way we're wired.

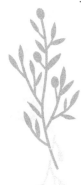

Early birds are apparently more proactive than evening people, and they tend to do well in business.

I always remind my patients that making the most of Early Risers Club means you need to join the "Early Bedtime Club" as well. It's also worth noting, however, that as we age, our sleep patterns are disrupted. We don't sleep as long, and we don't sleep as solidly as we did in our younger adult years.

So, what's the point of going to bed earlier and getting up earlier if your sleep is disrupted and unrestful? Well, as mentioned earlier, you have to stop covering up your issues with medication and instead start to address the root issues.

First, it's important to get testing done. You have to see where you may be dealing with issues that require treatment or a more aggressive approach. This includes hormones, adrenals, food sensitivities, nutritional deficiencies, a sleep study, and more.

Second, change your diet. I have seen time and time again—so many of my patients start to sleep better once they start to eat better. Digestion is an all-encompassing process for the body, and the Sinister Seven foods from Chapter Five can wreak havoc on your hormone balance and so much more. So, start eating better and see if you start to sleep better.

Third, consider adding supplements to your routine. We'll discuss a few of my favorite natural supplements at the end of this chapter.

Fourth, address your sleep hygiene. We'll do this next, and we'll also learn what a healthy sleep protocol looks like. It's not hard, but it will require some significant lifestyle adjustments, if you're doing nighttime like most of our fellow Americans. The term *sleep hygiene* is a variety of different practices and habits that are necessary to have good nighttime sleep quality and full daytime alertness.

These days, sleep hygiene is far more than using a noise machine, avoiding caffeine close to bedtime, or watching TV in bed.

The allopathic medicine world treats sleep much differently from those of us in the functional medicine world. In nursing school, I was taught to treat issues with sleep medications such as Ambien, which is a benzodiazepine. Tylenol PM and NyQuil are two other favorites in modern medicine. Basically, just after nursing school, when I heard the words "I can't sleep," that meant it was time to prescribe some pills.

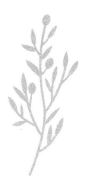

Sleeping pills are an inferior altnernative to finding out the real reason why you can't sleep.

That practice has failed you, and it has failed me. We have to *do* more and *dig* more.

In functional medicine, here are several of the steps I take in my office to make people more aware of proper sleep hygiene as well as get to the root cause of any sleeping disorder:

1. Take a thorough look at diet, lifestyle, relationships, past traumas, and more.

2. Talk about stress and its potential sources.

3. Emphasize the critical role of movement and exercise.

4. Work to limit screen time and EMF exposure.

5. Discuss what medications could be affecting your sleep.

6. Formulate a first-class nighttime protocol.

7. Consider some gentle nonpharmacological herbs, amino acids, magnesium, and others to help (but not become Band-Aid solutions).

8. Eliminate all caffeine after 3:00 p.m.

9. Figure out what kind of mattress you sleep on and if it's a help or a hindrance to a good night's rest.

10. Determine whether your spouse's or your own nighttime habits and/or snoring is affecting your sleep.

This is just the tip of the iceberg, and most people are frankly shocked to learn about all the things we do in our daily lives that prevent us from having a good night's sleep. Here are just a few examples of little things you may be doing that could be sabotaging your sleep:

* Going to bed at different times each night.

* Having stressful conversations in the evening just before bed.

* Not setting the temperature low enough (ideal temp is between 60 to 67 degrees).

* Drinking alcohol (despite what we've been told, "nightcaps" are terrible for sleep).

* Not getting enough sunlight during the early part of each day.

These are just a few. There are so many more! In the next section, you are going to learn that a healthy sleep protocol is maybe a little daunting but doable. For some, you may find it more palatable to incorporate a few of these pieces at a time and work toward creating your perfect sleep sanctuary.

Let's do this!

Dani's Wild & Well Sleep Protocol

Your bedroom needs to change. Right now, your bedroom is:

* The place where you watch TV.

* The area where you scroll through Instagram and Facebook.

* The setting where you and your spouse discuss finances after the kids go to bed.

* The go-to spot for munching on late-night snacks.

* Your favorite place to relax and sip on a glass of wine.

If you do any of these things now, it's okay. But let me tell you something that I tell every single one of my patients:

The bedroom is for sleep and sex only.

If you are not doing one of those two things, get out and come back when you are ready to get busy or get to sleep.

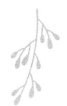

The bedroom is for sleep and sex only.

I tell my patients that sleep hygiene is just commonsense. The problem is that common sense is not so common anymore, is it? As we briefly touch on each point, just remember that this is all commonsense stuff—but, at the same time, it will require some minor and possibly less-than-minor lifestyle adjustments. But you can do it! So, here we go:

Prepare for sleep long before bed. About an hour before you plan to go to sleep, it's time to start winding down. Start thinking about going to bed and consciously slowing your pace and what you allow into your mind and take in through your senses. Don't watch programming that is going to give you negative thoughts (i.e., the news or anything violent, etc.) and watch the kinds of conversations in you get into in the hour or so before bed. Stressful conversations cause—you guessed it—a cortisol spike, and you want to avoid those as much as possible before bed.

Stop eating after dinner (with a caveat). Unless you have hypoglycemia (where your blood sugar drops in the night), you really have no reason to eat anything after dinner. I tell patients to stop eating after 7:00 p.m., whenever possible. If you are hypoglycemic, and you wake up in the night and can't go back to sleep, many times, that is a blood sugar problem. This could mean you are not consuming enough protein. So, I have those patients eat protein before they go to bed—as in a handful of nuts or a scoop of almond butter. You could also eat a small piece of chicken or drink a clean protein shake.

Skip the night cap. Alcohol does not help you sleep better at night. If you're going to drink, then drink a glass of wine with dinner (like the Europeans do). Europeans don't just drink to drink. They drink with food, and they're not day drinking on empty stomachs. Late night alcohol raises your blood sugar, and then it crashes your blood sugar between 2:00 and

4:00 a.m. When blood sugar crashes, guess what? Your cortisol levels go through the roof, and you wake up or just spend the rest of the night tossing and turning, only to wake up exhausted.

Bedtime matters. "Early to bed, early to rise" is a simple concept. If you want to get up early (around the time the sun comes up) and you need around seven or eight hours of sleep, you can do the math. You need to be going to bed by 10:00 p.m. So, pick a time and then stick with it every single night! Right now, if you are used to going to bed at midnight, try backing it up by fifteen minutes at a time every week or so. Every hour of sleep you get before midnight is worth two hours after midnight. We're designed to sleep at night when the moon is up and the sun is down. In fact, did you know that our eyesight is poor at night for a reason? We aren't designed to be able to peer into the darkness like night prowlers (lions, tigers, owls, etc.).

Keep it clean. Your bedroom should be neat and organized. When you walk into the room, think about the visual impact you want the room to convey to your psyche. If you see piles of unfolded clothes, you're going to feel pressured to fold them or at least feel guilty about *not* folding them. When you step across the threshold, make sure it whispers "sanctuary."

Soak it up. Take a bath and add some Epsom salts for added relaxation. Baths don't have to be an hour long. Even a fifteen-minute soak can do wonders for both your muscles and your mental state. Think about how great little kids sleep, and, most of the time, it's just after a long bath time. The hot water relaxes the muscles and provides a much-needed respite after a long day. I tell patients to add at least four cups of Epsom salts to the bath. The best way to absorb magnesium is trans-dermally.

Sip and relax. If you want to drink before bed, drink herbal teas like Sleepy Time, chamomile teas, valerian teas, or Holy Basil tea. Herbs that are designed to help promote relaxation are perfect to sip in place of alcohol or a caffeinated soda or acidic decaf coffee.

Tune the world out. If you want to scroll on social media or listen to the news, do it in the morning or at lunch. Just stop doing it at night! There is nothing on anyone's social media that you need to see at 9:00 p.m. Just relax and enjoy your own company or your partner's company. Enjoy some music before bed or put on some classical music while you read a good book or do a devotional with your spouse.

Have sex. I've said it before, but I'll say it again. If you are not having sex regularly with your spouse, you need to make a change. Kids and hectic careers *do* change everything, but sex doesn't have to be some long, drawn out process. However brief it needs to be, just make it happen. If you are a female, hear me now and hear me well. Your husband is not done with having sex, even if you feel you are. Find a way to feel sexy again and make this a part of your life! Your health and your marriage will both benefit.

Take off the watch. If you're one of those people who just HAS to track your sleep, get over it. Any benefit you gain from knowing your breakdown of light to deep sleep is negated by EMFs coursing through your body. If you really want to wear it, leave your Apple Watch or Fitbit in the bathroom and put it back on when you wake up. I used to sleep in my Fitbit every night, and since I stopped about two years ago, I noticed an improvement in my sleep and overall sense of feeling rested in the morning.

Get Fido his own bed. Pet owners, you may not want to hear this, but your fur babies need their own beds. People just don't sleep as well when they have animals all over them. Your dogs or cats toss and turn just like humans, and, oftentimes, our animals wake up in the middle of the night because they heard a noise or feel like playing (remember, they got to sleep all day, but you didn't). Get the animals out of your bedroom or, at the very least, out of your bed.

Work the day shift if possible. My patients who work in hospitals have crazy hours. I encourage every single one of them to put in for the day shift. Now, somebody's got to work the night shift, but the problem is that people who are chronic night shift workers tend to have shorter lives and more comorbidities.[240] We're not designed to be up all night. If you do have to work at night and sleep during the day, make sure you have some high-quality blackout curtains that block out ALL light and use a soothing noise machine in your room. White noise is nice, but also check out green and brown noise. They have deeper frequencies, and many people prefer them to the shriller white noise.

Activate night mode. If you are looking at your phone close to bedtime, make sure it is on "night mode" where the blue light is filtered out. The electric glow from your phone doesn't do your body any favors, particular at night when the setting sun is supposed to trigger our bodies to get ready for sleep and repair time. I also recommend that you watch TV through blue light filter glasses—but don't use them during the day because they suppress the bright light signal, which could interfere with alertness and confuse the light/dark circadian signals.[241]

Do a sleep study. If either you or your spouse snores, that person needs a sleep study. There are home studies, but one conducted in a lab is ideal for better accuracy. A pulmonologist friend of mine, Dr. Bill Noah, once told me, "Untreated sleep apnea takes ten to sixteen years off of your lifespan." So, don't take it for granted, and make sure you know what you are dealing with.

Move bedrooms if necessary. If your spouse does snore, you may need to move bedrooms. Your body heals when you sleep, and if you are constantly being awakened by the sound of snoring, your body will suffer as a result. My patients who switch to another bedroom in the house report that both their health *and* their marriage are better. You can always "visit" your spouse's bed or vice versa. When I was young, I remember asking my grandma about how she felt about sleeping in a different bed than my granddaddy since she slept in another room due to his horrible snoring. She smiled and said, "Oh, Dani, I go across and visit Granddaddy whenever I need to." I had no idea what that meant at the time, but I'll never forget the day many years later when I realized she was talking about having sex with my granddaddy.

Say no to electromagnetic fields. And now for our final element of my Wild & Well Sleep Protocol: dealing with the giant elephant in the bedroom… electricity. This topic is so important that it needs its own section. So, here we go.

Sound Sleep and EMFs Just Don't Mix

Do you sleep on a sleep number bed? If so, I have some bad news for you. You need to think about finding a replacement. Our bodies weren't meant to sleep on top of an electricity mine field.

Do you lay your phone on your bed to track your sleep or leave it plugged in and charging beside your bed? Well, then, I also have some bad news for you. You need to get away from your phone at night—far, far away. Airplane mode is great, but if it's plugged in to an outlet within six feet of your head, airplane mode is not doing any good because you're getting still those EMFs from the outlet.

So, what exactly are EMFs? EMF stands for electromagnetic field. And EMFs are present everywhere in our environment but are invisible to the human eye. There are natural sources of EMFs, such as those caused by the earth's magnetic field and the local build-up of electric charges in the atmosphere associated with thunderstorms.

Then there are the man-made versions such as x-rays the low frequency electromagnetic fields associated with each and every power socket and powered device in your home. There are also higher frequency radio waves that are used to transmit information via TV antennas, radio stations, and cellphone towers.

Simply plugging a wire into an outlet creates electric fields in the air surrounding that device or appliance. The higher the voltage, the stronger the field produced. And it doesn't even matter if the appliance is on or off. The voltage exists even when no current is flowing.

EMFs are no good for our bodies. This has been proven in literally thousands of studies. I could write a whole book on EMFs and probably will because I believe so strongly in helping people heal from the years of EMF exposure that we willingly undergo each and every day. EMF exposure has been linked to cancer, autoimmune diseases, reduced immune function, depression, weight gain, and so much more.[242,243,244]

Many people don't realize that they have an extreme sensitivity to EMFs. Here are just a few of the side effects of EMF sensitivity or prolonged exposure:[245]

- Skin symptoms such as facial prickling, burning sensations, and rashes

- Body symptoms such as muscular aches and pains

- Fatigue, stress, and sleep disturbances

- Eye symptoms such as burning and itching

- Neurological symptoms such as brain fog thinking and depression

- Ear, nose, and throat symptoms

- Digestive disorders

- Infertility

- Leukemia in children, breast cancer, and other cancers (in some cases)

Even if they don't have an actual condition like electromagnetic hypersensitivity (EHS), I still tell my patients to unplug everything around their beds. This includes any adjustable bed platforms, lamps, and phone charging stations. If you use your phone as your alarm clock, move it all the way across the bedroom or, better yet, across the hall. You can do what I do:

> **Get an old-fashioned alarm clock with batteries and set that beside the bed. Whatever you do, just get that phone away from your bed now!**

Get an old-fashioned alarm clock with batteries and set that beside the bed. Whatever you do, just get that phone away from your bed now!

Is your wireless router located in your bedroom? Move it elsewhere. Experts say that there has to be a minimum of two walls between your bedroom and your wireless router.

Is there a TV, cable box, or computer in your bedroom? You guessed it—get that mess out of your sleep sanctuary.

Even if you have a CPAP machine for sleep apnea, I tell my OSA patients to plug it in out in the hallway and get an extension cord. Whatever you can do to unplug everything in your bedroom, make it happen.

Do you have a baby monitor right beside your baby's crib with wireless technology? Get that stuff away from your little bundle and let that precious angel sleep without all the EMF interference.

We're around EMFs all day long at work and in our busy lives. The least we can do is give our bodies a rest from it at night. I have a whole lot more information on the dangers of EMFs in my Sunday Night Services that are available on YouTube (YouTube channel: Dani Williamson Wellness) and on my website, **DaniWilliamson.com**. If you'd like to find out more, dig in and learn how to avoid the damaging effects of EMFs for you and your family.

Remember, your bedroom should be a serene sleep and sex sanctuary! If it's not, start making some changes and notice the dramatic improvement in both your health and your marriage.

Supplements that Support Sleep

I tell everyone I know that if you aren't eating well, there's a good chance you aren't sleeping well. And if you aren't moving well, pooping well, connecting well, and especially relaxing well, you are depriving yourself of good sleep.

Supplements are not a replacement for these key elements, but if you are doing your best in the other areas and still need some help, a supplement or two could be the key for you.

If you are taking any medications for sleep, speak with a functional medical professional before starting any new supplements, and remember that not everything works for everyone. Here are a few supplements to discuss with your doctor.

CBD OIL

I'm a big believer in cannabidiol, or CBD oil. I have experienced firsthand and heard from countless patients that it is phenomenal for sleep, particularly for those who can go to sleep fairly easily but have trouble *staying* asleep. CBD oil is a relative newcomer to the sleep space, but there is already a slew of research to support its use to help you get a good night's rest. Always make sure you take a full spectrum, third-party tested, CO_2 critically extracted, organic CBD oil (and watch out for the snake oil that has flooded the market).

5-HTP

5-Hydroxytryptophan (5-HTP) is a phenomenal sleep aid. Also known as oxitriptan, 5-HTP is a naturally occurring amino acid and chemical precursor as well as a metabolic intermediate in the production of serotonin. Tryptophan converts to 5-HTP, 5-HTP converts to serotonin, and serotonin converts to melatonin. I recommend 100 to 200 milligrams of 5-HTP. Take it with a B vitamin for even more benefit. One side effect of 5-HTP is that it decreases carbohydrate and sugar cravings—and that's never a bad thing.

VITAMIN D

Micronutrients and sleep patterns and disorders are linked. One of the micronutrient deficiencies that wreak havoc on the body is vitamin D deficiency. If you aren't getting ample sunlight during the day (first thing in the morning is the best time to get some sunshine), then you may need to use a supplement. Always find your Vitamin D3 level before starting supplementation.

MAGNESIUM

Experts say that up to 80 percent of the adult population is deficient in magnesium. Sometimes, all my patients need is 300 to 500 milligrams of magnesium glycinate chelate, and they start to sleep like they haven't slept in years. Simple as that. Their restless legs go away, and they sleep like never before. If you struggle with calming down at night, you may have a magnesium deficiency. When in doubt, get tested and know for sure!

TRYPTOPHAN

I suggest tryptophan for many patients who have a lot of anxiety. Tryptophan works beautifully at 500 milligrams twice a day, afternoon and evening. Tryptophan is a precursor to serotonin and it's the ingredient in turkey that makes you feel so sleepy on Thanksgiving. 5-HTP converts to tryptophan, and tryptophan converts to serotonin in our bodies. When serotonin is low, you may experience insomnia, anxiety, and depression. If you're taking anti-depressants, ask your provider if you can take tryptophan.

MELATONIN

Even though it's been used for years and approved to be safe for kids, melatonin is a hormone some mistakenly believe will disrupt their own production of melatonin. The research does not show that. In fact, melatonin is anti-inflammatory and anti-viral (which is why it's part of hospital protocols for Covid-19 patients), and it decreases oxidative stress in the body while helping you sleep. Dr Lindsey Berkson is an expert on melatonin, and she and I have a video on our YouTube channel on the benefits of melatonin. She even uses it with breast cancer patients. Some people don't like melatonin, citing that it causes bizarre dreams and insomnia. I have never experienced this and personally take 3 milligrams (immediate release) at night. If you have trouble going to sleep, take immediate release (IR), if you have trouble staying asleep take controlled release (CR). If you struggle with both, then take both IR and CR. Start with a low dosage (0.5 mg) and increase as needed.

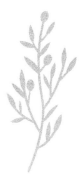

Other fantastic herbs that help promote sound sleep are lemon balm, holy basil, and valerian.

ASHWAGANDHA

Ashwagandha is unbelievable for sleep. It is an adaptogen (an herb that restores balance and provides stabilization) that works to bring cortisol levels into proper balance and helps you go to sleep. Taking 250 to 350 milligrams at bedtime works well for many people. The botanical name for Ashwagandha is *withania somnifera*, which means sleep! Ashwagandha is in the nightshade family, which means if you are sensitive to nightshades, you may want to skip this herb.

Other fantastic herbs that help promote sound sleep are lemon balm, holy basil, and valerian.

PROGESTERONE

Progesterone is a game changer for sleep. Progesterone is your calming hormone and the hormone that decreases PMS and breast tenderness. It's also the very first hormone that starts to decrease in your early thirties.

Progesterone, for many women, is the golden ticket to great sleep.

I started progesterone when I was 44 and saw an immediate improvement in my sleep. Every time I have my hormone levels checked, my progesterone levels are perfect. That is why I adamantly suggest that you get tested and do it right. Don't mess with your hormones, especially not this key hormone.

I am a huge fan of bioidentical progesterone, either via a cream or taken orally.

Some people sleep better with oral progesterone that is compounded by any certified compounding pharmacy (you don't want just anybody making your hormones).

Transdermal progesterone creams are great and some doctors prefer transdermal over oral progesterone due to the systemic absorption. Many of my perimenopausal patients tell me they also notice a dramatic improvement in their sleep when they start using progesterone.

Progesterone, for many women, is the golden ticket to great sleep.

Progesterone is not just a "helpful" supplement; it's something that the vast majority of my aging female patients need. Many women tell me they slept beautifully until menopause. That was me. I slept like a log my whole life, even when my kids were little. Then I turned 49 and everything changed. That is the year then my hormones really started shifting and menopause began.

Unlike with progesterone, other sleep aids and sleep supplements act as Band-Aids rather than address a deficiency. Your body is not deficient in Ambien or even CBD oil. Use supplements as needed but never stop digging to find the root cause of your sleep issues!

Don't Mess with Sleep

Your body heals when you sleep. It is as simple and as complicated as that right there. If you don't sleep well, you can't heal—and you can't decrease inflammation. You won't be able to lose the weight, your stress levels will stay high, and you just won't be able to shake that feeling of exhaustion.

Every adult needs between seven to nine hours of sleep. Prove me wrong. I'll wait.

The end results could very well be disease and years taken off your lifespan.

Few (if any) people are able to operate well on five hours of sleep a night. If anyone tells you they are "fine" with six or fewer hours of shut-eye, they are kidding themselves or in denial. Our bodies regenerate, recirculate, and recalculate completely when we sleep.

Every adult needs between seven to nine hours of sleep. Prove me wrong. I'll wait.

Follow the Wild & Well Sleep Protocol in this chapter and get the proper testing to see if you are dealing with a hormonal imbalance, adrenal issue, or nutritional deficiency.

Don't eat after dinner, unplug everything in your bedroom, and turn it into a sex and sleep sanctuary.

Meditate and pray in the evenings, and find the calm amidst the storms of life long enough to allow your body to relax and slip into much-needed unconsciousness.

If you do not sleep well, you will not be well.

Did you know that just one night of sleep deprivation can increase insulin resistance? Don't mess with your sleep! Just give your body what it needs to thrive by getting those *zzzs*!

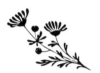

wild & well Rx
Dani Williamson, MSN, FNP

R

Patient Name: ....

Age: ....   Date: ....

1. Get out of the bed if you aren't sleeping or having sex.

2. Give yourself lots grace if you don't sleep through the night. Remember, the first and second sleeps that have disappeared throughout the centuries.

3. Pay attention to how you feel when you wake up, midday, afternoon, and in the evening.

4. Consider weaning off sleep prescriptions and replacing them with better habits and sleep hygiene.

5. Transform your bedroom into a sanctuary—a place that says 'sleep well' when you cross its threshold.

6. Get your sleep hygiene routine nailed down and don't miss it!

7. Go to a sleep center ASAP to be evaluated for sleep apnea if you snore.

8. Move to a different bedroom if partner/spouse snores. You can get together for some intimate time and then sleep soundly!

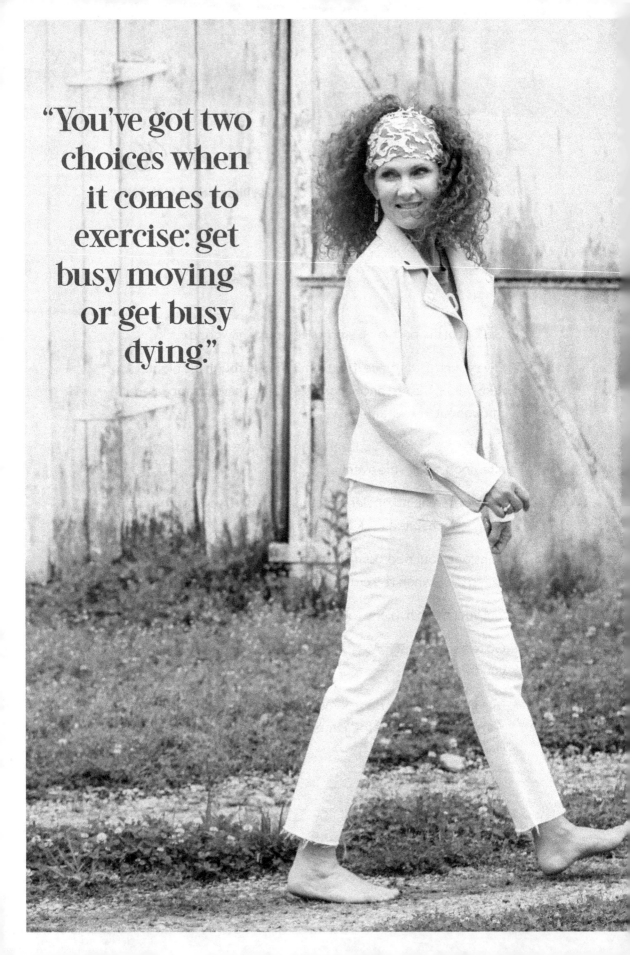

"You've got two choices when it comes to exercise: get busy moving or get busy dying."

move well

*"If swimming is such a good way to stay in shape,
explain whales."*

UNKNOWN

At this point in society, with all of the information about health and fitness that we have available to us instantly on our phones, on our computers, and on the TV…

- With 24-hour gyms on every corner…

- With boutique fitness studios popping up like hotcakes…

- With celebrities and their six-packs and toned legs on Instagram…

- With Apple watches tracking our every step…

- With CrossFit and Orangetheory and every other trend before them…

- With Facebook marketing the latest HIIT workout on our feeds 24/7…

- With apps that give us libraries of workouts at our fingertips…

… we all know by now that movement is important.

Right? I certainly hope so.

Our bodies are designed to move, and they don't work as well when we don't. It really is as simple as that. However, for those who still need a little more convincing, we're going to briefly discuss the extreme importance of moving your body in an intentional way—and how downright fun it can become.

A decline in movement is linked to a decline in longevity, and unless you've got a goal to not outlive your friends and family, then you need to re-think the number of minutes that you spend being active every day.

It's not necessarily your fault that it now takes so much intentional effort to move. Life used to be much more naturally conducive to movement. It wasn't until about 100 years ago that life became a whole lot more sedentary for a whole lot of people—and pretty rapidly.

In 1908, the Ford Model T began production and, from 1913 to 1927, Ford mass produced the first 15 million cars, thanks to Henry Ford's handy-dandy assembly line. Still, there were over 100 million people in the U.S. at the time, so plenty of folks were still walking.

But that all changed for good soon after. Once the average family was able to afford a car, more people could move to the suburbs, and American cities became sprawling metropolises that were impossible to traverse on foot or even on bike.

People no longer walked to school or walked to the corner market for the goods they needed.

The death of family-owned farms, the birth of corporate farms and food plants, and the rise of chain grocery stores further impacted human movement. People didn't have to grow their own food anymore. They could just park in a space right in front of a giant store filled with food.

So simple! So convenient!

Such a disaster when it came to bodies staying in motion.

Then there are TVs, video games, and, of course, our beloved smart phones.

Kids once went outside to play ball but now are content to "play" with virtual friends on a screen.

As for the rest of us—in the morning, on lunch break, and after dinner, grown adults are choosing to stay trapped behind their little electric rectangles and scroll through social media rather than going for a walk with the family, throwing the ball around in the backyard, or playing tag with the kids.

We're getting fatter, but we're moving less. How much sense does that make?

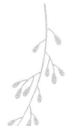

We're getting fatter, but we're moving less. How much sense does that make?

We sit on the same inviting and familiar indent on the couch cushion night after night as we stuff our faces, and then we actually have the audacity to wonder why we don't feel well. A lot of it is habit. If your family's nightly routine involves watching TV, that is just what you do. If your habit is scrolling through social media in your spare time, that is just what you do.

But does it have to stay that way?

Sadly, it usually does until you get a wake-up call. Maybe your doctor tells you that you're pre-diabetic. Maybe your blood pressure has been steadily increasing over the last decade and now it's in dangerous territory.

Humans are pretty consistent, and we also usually wait for some sort of crisis before we decide to change our habits.

I'm not condemning modern life (okay, maybe I am), but I will say that it has made it so that if you want to move, you have to plan to move.

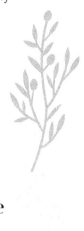

I'm not condemning modern life, but I will say that it has made it so that if you want to move, you have to plan to move.

It turns out lots of people aren't really buying into this truth. As a result, we now have horrible statistics, like the ones listed on the following page, to contend with:

- Almost 32 percent of children and adolescents are either overweight or obese.[246]

- Close to 20 percent of children and adolescents aged 2 to 19 years in the U.S. are actually considered obese.[247]

- Cardiovascular disease continues to be the leading cause of death in the U.S., despite the knowledge that those who adhere to commonsense guidelines for a healthful diet and physical activity have lower rates of cardiovascular morbidity and mortality than those who do not.[248]

- Only 23.2 percent of adults aged 18 and over are able to meet the "Physical Activity Guidelines" for both aerobic and muscle-strengthening activity.[249]

Here is the bottom line, folks. There is conclusive and overwhelming evidence that physical inactivity is one of the most significant causes of most chronic diseases.

As an extension of that, there is evidence to show that activity, movement, exercise, or whatever else you want to call it is one of the absolute best ways to prevent at least thirty-five of the most common chronic conditions and diseases. That list includes:[250]

- Accelerated biological aging/premature death and age-associated pain

- Metabolic syndrome and obesity

- Insulin resistance, pre-diabetes, and type 2 diabetes

- Nonalcoholic fatty liver disease

- Coronary heart disease, peripheral artery disease, hypertension, stroke, congestive heart failure, hemostasis, and deep vein thrombosis

- Cognitive dysfunction, depression and anxiety

- Osteoporosis, osteoarthritis, balance, bone fracture/falls, and rheumatoid arthritis

- Colon cancer, breast cancer, and endometrial cancer

- Gestational diabetes and pre-eclampsia

- Polycystic ovary syndrome and erectile dysfunction

- Diverticulitis, constipation, and gallbladder diseases

Will a gym membership be enough to thwart many of these conditions and stay active? For some, yes. For many others, that's a resounding no. Over half of all Americans pay for a gym membership they do not use, and this amounts for a whopping $1.8 billion on unused gym memberships.[251] That's just ludicrous!

If you are one of those people who joins the gym every year after your New Year's resolution to "lose weight" or "get healthy" but never goes, you can rest easy. I'm not going to tell you to join the gym. You already know if you're a "gym person," and if you aren't, why waste the money on a membership?

Many of my fittest, healthiest friends have never been members of any gym. You don't have to go to a gym to be fit and healthy. Exercise is simple. So, we'll spend the rest of this chapter discussing the best "hacks" for those who are less inclined to work out than others. If you happen to be a regular at the gym already or are an avid runner, good for you! Keep reading, because I have some words of advice and tips for you as well.

Make Movement Instinctive

I tell my patients all the time, "You have to make movement a part of your everyday life." So many of us have sedentary jobs. I am in my office for most of the day talking to patients. On the surface, that sounds pretty unhealthy, being stuck inside all day. That is why I know that if you are inside for the majority of the day like I am, you've got to shake things up and keep that body in motion, someway and somehow!

Does that mean you should go workout in the morning for an hour before work or spend two hours after work on a run? If those options sound fun to you, then yes! But those aren't the only choices.

Interestingly, in a study of two groups of powerlifters conducted in Norway, "group one" trained once a day, while "group two" did the exact same program but split into two parts—half in the morning and half in the evening.[252]

The results clearly showed that group two made *superior gains in every way* over group one. The two-a-day group was able to lift significantly more weight despite the fact that both groups did the exact same routine and exercises with the same total volume and intensity.

> ## Get that blood pumping and move every single hour.

The takeaway from a study like that is that *longer* does not automatically equal *better* when it comes to a workout. "Do what you can, when you can" wins all day long over "do nothing at all," and in many cases, it even beats, "work out until exhaustion."

How long does it take to do ten squats—maybe 30 seconds? What if you stood up every 30 minutes to an hour and did a few squats? You'd easily fit 100 squats into your day without really even trying!

Get that blood pumping and move every single hour.

Don't make excuses. Just do it.

You can do a quick set of crunches or bicep curls in between phone calls, in between clients, or in between meetings. If you work from home, stop what you are doing every hour or so and run up and down the stairs a few times. Let's say you are helping your kids with their schoolwork. While they are writing something down, do some pushups or burpees.

Working out doesn't have to be something that you stop your life to do, perform faithfully for an hour or more, and then go back to life (you can do it that way, if you prefer, but it's not a requirement). Instead, make movement a frequent and recurring part of your daily life and encourage your kids to do the same! Here are a few other ways to incorporate movement into your routine:

- Place your palms on the kitchen counter and do a few pushups while you're cooking.

- Hop down into a plank while you are waiting for the water on the stove to boil.

- Do jumping jacks before you sit down for dinner. Better yet, have the whole family do them with you! The family that moves together is healthier together.

- Do bicep curls with your grocery bags as you carry them inside.

- Use your iron skillets to do triceps extensions.

The list is endless!

I personally love my stand-up desk at work. When I have to spend time in front of my computer or do paperwork, I do it standing up and moving my legs. I have worked way too hard to restore my health to spend all day sitting on my butt!

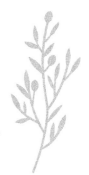

Make movement a frequent and recurring part of your daily life and encourage your kids to do the same!

There are some pretty inventive products on the market to help you keep moving at work. There are sleek treadmills that fit under a desk. Combine one of those with a stand-up desk, and you can walk all day long (just be sure to choose a pace you can maintain without watching your feet). There are also mini stair steppers that you can place under your stand-up desk, as well as cycles that you can use while seated.

If you have a gym membership that you don't ever use, cancel it and use the money you are saving to buy one of these amazing pieces of equipment to help keep you moving during the day.

There are so many ways to exercise for free. You don't need a $2,000

Peloton bike to be fit and healthy. I read a story about a woman who literally ran a marathon inside her home during the 2020 quarantine! If she can do that, you can find the time and a way to work out, both at home and at work.

Yoga is Life

If there was one activity that I believe deserves its own intentional time every week, it would be yoga. There's a reason the practice of yoga has been around for thousands of years. It works, and, boy, does it do a body good.

Boutique gyms and the latest trendy workouts? A workout is all well and good if that is what gets you the results you need *and* doesn't deplete you or exhaust your adrenals—but keep in mind that those types of exercises haven't been around for millennia. They also haven't been studied long enough to fully understand any potential long-term repercussions.

If you exercise and you feel worse afterwards (your endorphins may be pumping and you feel better mentally, but you have to go home and take a two-hour nap), then you're doing the wrong exercise.

Healthy adrenals are one of the keys to ensuring that you have an energetic, productive day. And as much as avid fitness enthusiasts may not want to admit it, not every hard workout is as beneficial in the long run as it seems on the surface.

If you feel truly depleted after a workout, it may not be the right workout, plain and simple. On the other hand, I've yet to meet a single person who wouldn't benefit from doing yoga.

If your workout burns a thousand calories but you're toast afterwards— well, all I can say is there is more to movement than calories burned. I've had plenty of women tell me that they kill themselves at the gym, in cycle classes, or running mile after mile, and they still don't lose the kind of weight they thought they would. This could be because strenuous exercise increases inflammation in the body, and if it's a daily process, there could be unintended consequences.

All I'm asking you to do is listen to your body. Give it what it really needs, not what your friends are doing or what you think it needs based on an Instagram story you saw last month.

If you are always getting injured, always seem to be icing a pulled muscle, or continually suffer from aching joints as a result of your activities, it may be time to consider giving your body some other options.

High intensity activity is just not meant for some people. But yoga? The development of yoga can be traced back over five thousand years.

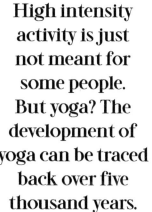

High intensity activity is just not meant for some people. But yoga? The development of yoga can be traced back over five thousand years.

Some researchers think that yoga even may be as much as ten thousand years old. The earliest forms of yoga can be found in the most ancient sacred texts known to mankind.

Yoga teaches you about breath and breath control, or pranayama. Pranayama means *life force*, and without breath, you don't have any life in your body. Purposefully filling your lungs with oxygen and exhaling and then controlling that process is one of the most beneficial things you can do for your lungs, your heart, your stress levels, and your state of mind.

In many studies, researchers have concluded that in both healthy and diseased populations, yoga may be as effective as or *better* than exercise at improving a variety of health-related outcome measures.[253] The reason cited for yoga's superior results is the proven fact that yoga benefits both physical *and* mental health via down-regulation of the hypothalamic–pituitary–adrenal (HPA) axis and the sympathetic nervous system (SNS).[254] In other words:

Yoga is great for your brain, your mood, and your stress levels!

If you have never practiced yoga, I highly encourage you to give it a try. I even recommend it to my male patients, many of whom scoff at the idea— that is, until they actually try it and are sore for a week afterwards!

Some Christians are bothered by the spiritual aspects of yoga. I won't argue about where yoga was founded and by whom it was traditionally practiced and why, but I look at it like I look at a Christmas tree. Most Christians know that the Christmas tree has pagan roots, right? Wait a minute—you mean that we celebrate the birth of Jesus Christ using pagan symbols? We sure do.

> **Yoga is great for your brain, your mood, and your stress levels!**

The same thing happens at Easter every time your kids go on an Easter egg hunt.

I hope you get my point here.

This world we live in and the things we do almost without thinking anymore are all watered down by centuries of diverse cultures and assorted beliefs intermingling. Now, if you don't put up a Christmas tree out of principle, then I understand it if you also don't want to practice yoga. For me, however, yoga is simply a superior form of healthy physical exercise, and it also provides me with additional time to pray and meditate on the Bible.

When in doubt, ask God for discernment and do what is right for *you*. It's been years since I've even been in a studio that pushes the spiritual side of yoga. Find a yoga teacher (through an online course, an app, DVDs, YouTube, or a local studio) who helps you get the most physical benefits out of yoga, and you may also discover a reinvigoration of your prayer life during the quiet moments of your practice.

There are so many great yoga programs that you can do at home for free or a small fee, or you can join a yoga studio if you have room in your budget for that (most boutique studios range from $100 to $200 for monthly memberships where you can work out several times a week). Many of my patients swear by hot yoga, where you practice in higher temps and therefore sweat a lot more. I taught yoga for years in a heated room and love hot yoga with a vinyasa flow. Whatever you choose, make sure you will stick to it.

Your body *craves* being stretched, so give it what it wants through an ancient exercise with proven health benefits, and you'll enjoy longer, leaner muscles in the process.

Move It or Lose It

As we age, our bodies age with us (I know, hard to believe, right?). One day, you wake up and look in the mirror, and that college-age kid you feel like inside looks like someone you used to call "super old" when you were younger.

Like it or not, we're all going to get old. Frankly, it's a blessing! After all, what's the alternative?

However, one less desirable part of aging is the fact that with each passing year, we feel stiffer and less bendy. It's a little bit like we're the Tinman from *The Wizard of Oz*. As we age, we tend to slow down, and, after a while, our old "nuts and bolts" just sort of start to rust over and feel stuck.

The harsh truth is that unless you want to feel like the Tinman every time you wake up in the morning or get up from the recliner, you're going to have to move—and move a lot.

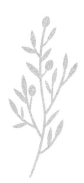

> **Moderate weight-bearing exercise was identified as a protective factor with regard to bone loss.**

As we age, our skeletal mass also starts to decrease, and this makes our bones more brittle (hence, why grandma's fall broke her hip, but little Billy can fall off the monkey bars and laugh as he climbs back up again). The degree of *osteopenia*, or low bone mass, you will experience depends on two things: 1) nutritional status, as in sufficient amounts of calcium, vitamin D, protein, etc., and 2) exercise.[255]

And not just any type of exercise. The focus should be on low-impact and weight bearing movements. In a study of 40 healthy people over the age of 50, researchers showed that extreme levels of exercise (which amounted to about 45 minutes a day of strenuous activity, seven days a week) actually caused bone density to decrease![256] Yikes. On the other hand:

Moderate weight-bearing exercise was identified as a protective factor with regard to bone loss.

In another study, resistance training was shown to have a positive effect on multiple risk factors for osteoporotic fractures in previously sedentary, post-menopausal women.[257] Especially as you age, you need to show your body some love through low-impact but challenging cardio and weight bearing movement.

No weights? No problem! Lift some cans of beans or broth over your head for a few minutes a day. Do bicep curls with a grandchild or your dog. You gotta use it or you're gonna lose it!

Looking for something to do but not interested in going to a gym filled with young, firm bodies? Try ballroom dancing! When you learn the dance steps, it takes a lot to remember them and perform them in the proper order and in time to the music. You also have to be spatially aware of your partner. So, your brain is forced to get a workout, and this keeps you sharp and really helps fire up the neural pathways in the brain. What I love most about ballroom dancing is that it has been documented to help with Parkinson's and cognitive disorders such as Alzheimer's.

- **Dancing for Parkinson's.** In studies, ballroom dances such as the tango may benefit both balance and locomotion, which can help lessen the symptoms of Parkinson's.[258]

- **Dancing for Alzheimer's**. In another study, 129 elderly patients with amnestic mild cognitive impairment (aMCI) were divided into two groups. One group took ballroom dancing for ten months, while the other group was sedentary. Both groups were subjected to extensive neuropsychological assessment prior to and after the ten-month period. The results were amazing. The dancing group showed significant improvements on the tests, while the other group's results got worse. They concluded that ballroom dancing can positively impact cognitive function.[259]

I tell my young patients daily that youth is forgiving—but you *will* reach an age in life when you may very well wake up with an unexplained "sleeping injury." There may come a time when you look back at someone behind you and throw out your neck. These are just some of the occupational hazards of aging.

Growing old gracefully isn't for sissies. You have to put the work in. If you don't, the outcomes could be pain, more pain, stiffness, reduced sleep quality, weight gain, mood disorders, cardiovascular disease, and much more.

If you are young now, don't wait until you're older to start moving. And if you're older, don't wait another day. Put this book down right now and go for a brisk walk.

The easiest way to work out is just to start.

Put on your shoes and walk out the door. Find a yoga workout on YouTube and do some stretches right there in your living room. There are workouts designed for each and every fitness level, somewhere out there. There are workouts for people with back issues, knee issues, weight issues, you name it. So, there are no excuses to stay motionless that will work anymore.

When I think of the personification of exercizse and fitness, I don't even think of a youthful, beautiful person like Giselle Bundchen or a Kardashian, or even a modern pro athlete like Serena Williams.

> **When I think of fitness, my mind always goes to Jack LaLanne, also known as The Godfather of Fitness.**

When I think of fitness, my mind always goes to Jack LaLanne, also known as The Godfather of Fitness.

For those of you who are old enough to remember this legend, let's reminisce together. For those who have never heard of him, take a moment to learn from the best. Born in 1914, Jack was a self-described "'junk food junkie" until, as a teen, he attended a lecture by health pioneer Dr. Paul Bragg on the importance of a healthy diet. His life would never be the same after that lecture. He went on to write many books on health and also hosted the longest-running TV fitness show of all time, "The Jack LaLanne Show," from 1953 to 1985.

Jack had some key habits that he practiced faithfully and preached daily to others for decades. Here are just a few of the things he did regularly:

* **Early to bed, early to rise.** Jack got up early. More specifically, he was up by 4:00 a.m. in his younger years and by 5:00 a.m. to 6:00 a.m. later in life.

- **Stretch to start the day.** He stretched in bed before he even put his feet on the ground.

- **Work out before breakfast.** Jack exercised first thing in the morning before he ate breakfast. He is said to have never missed his morning workout because he wanted to "earn his breakfast."

- **Keep the body guessing.** One of his fundamental principles was to keep the body guessing and never fall into a predictable exercise routine. He was known to regularly switch up his routine in order to keep his muscles from adapting.

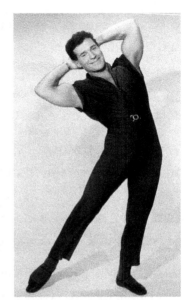

- **Don't skip cardio.** Although Jack was definitely a bodybuilder, he understood the importance of cardio for heart health and, therefore, considered it to be just as important as weight training.

- **Lift like you mean it.** He lifted to failure. Jack lifted an amount of weight that he could only carry out for anywhere from ten to fifteen reps of any given exercise.

- **Swim for the win.** Jack felt that swimming was the most superior form of cardiovascular exercise because it's not just low but zero impact, works all the major muscle groups, vastly improves overall endurance, and also helps posture and flexibility.

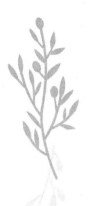

> "You have 640 muscles in the human body. I take every one of them into account as I plan an exercise routine."
>
> JACK LALANNE

Jack worked out in these one-piece jumpsuits that were his signature look and not something that most of us would be caught dead in—but somehow, they worked for him. He died at age 96 after a bout of pneumonia, but it's reported that he performed his daily workout routine right up until the day he passed away.

Isn't that incredible?

This man represented all that is good about exercise, and what I love most is he always kept it simple—he recommended such straightforward exercises like jumping jacks, pushups, sit ups, and even running in place.

He was also way ahead of his time when it came to diet. He talked frequently about the dangers of white sugar, white flour, and alcohol—and this was way back in in the 60s and 70s!

Jack LaLanne used common sense, and that is something we need a whole lot more of these days. If you are sick and tired of being sick and tired, and diet alone isn't cutting it, then you need to start moving!

You can choose to stay active all day (and you can even wear a one-piece jumpsuit if you feel like it).

> "If man made it, don't eat it."
> JACK LALANNE

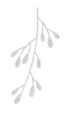

You don't have to join CrossFit or Gold's or Pure Barre or Buti Yoga. There is nothing you need to do other than just get up and move your body every day. And frankly, would it be so bad if you went for a 30- to 45-minute brisk walk in the evening with your partner? Get that heartrate up and move it—and spend some quality and probably much-needed time with your partner or spouse.

It's time to get back to the basics, and that is what Jack LaLanne was all about. Nothing fancy. Just free, effective movement that helps you live longer and feel better. Let's stop over-complicating this, because trying to figure out the exact number of minutes you should keep your heartrate at a certain rate is frankly just too much for most people.

> "Would you give your dog a cigarette and a donut for breakfast every morning?"
> JACK LALANNE

I don't know about you, but I think we need a little more of Jack LaLanne's principles in our lives. Strip away all the fluff and fancy terms and just get back to what works. Set a goal to do some form of non-jarring cardio and weight bearing exercises at least three to four days a week, especially as you age.

#KeepItSimpleSis #KeepItSimpleSir

Dani's Wild & Well Exercise Success Habits

We've already discussed so many little hacks and ways to incorporate more movement into your daily routines, as well as the reasons why doing so is of the utmost importance to your health. As we near the end of the chapter, I want to give you three other keys to making exercise a part of who you are:

1. FIND A WORKOUT BUDDY.

If you struggle to find the motivation to work out, find someone to work out alongside you. Even those of us who enjoy working out have days when we just don't want to move. That's when a workout buddy comes in handy.

Exercising with a good friend or even just an acquaintance is one way to hold yourself accountable. It's almost impossible to skip out on your morning workout when you have someone waiting outside for you at 5:00 a.m. in the cold.

If you are a competitive person like I am, you will find that a little friendly competition really helps you increase your intensity. There is no way that I am going to let my friend jog faster than me on that treadmill! Just note that if you are competitive, then you need to make sure that you pick a partner who has similar physical abilities to yours. That way you don't push yourself beyond your limits or vice versa.

2. WORK OUT IN THE MORNING.

We talked a lot about squeezing in your workout whenever you can during the day. That is definitely better than not working out at all, but when it comes to timing, the research shows that working out in the morning is the absolute best thing you can do for your body.

A morning workout is ideal for matching your body's hormonal fluctuations—and, in particular, your cortisol production. As we have discussed previously, cortisol (aka the stress hormone) is the hormone that keeps you awake and alert. Cortisol increases in the morning and drops in the evening, and it reaches its peak around 9:00 a.m. Therefore, your body might be more prime to move during peak cortisol production.

Additionally, morning activity may give you a much-needed mood boost. During exercise, your brain produces more *endorphins*, or the feel-good neurotransmitters. You will feel a sense of accomplishment, and your day will start on a more positive note with some movement in the morning.

Early workouts are also best for weight loss. In one study, ten male patients exercised in the morning, afternoon, and evening over separate sessions. Researchers found that the men stayed in fat-burning mode for the longest when they exercised in the morning before the first meal of the day.[260] So, if you're looking to lose some weight, morning exercise may just be the thing you need.

3. FIND THE MOTIVATION TO MOVE.

Finding the motivation to move is everything. So, where does it come from and how can you find more of it? I don't have that answer for you, because that comes from deep inside each person. Do some soul searching to find what motivation is to you.

For some, the motivation may be bikini season. For others, they could care less about how they look in a swimsuit. Some people are simply looking to not be in pain when going up the stairs.

- Maybe there is a little black dress you have your eye on.

- Maybe you want to sleep better.

- Maybe you want to reverse pre-diabetes and get your numbers normal.

- Maybe you want to make sure you are still alive to meet your grandkids.

- Find your WHY... and then make it happen.

Whatever your why may be, you absolutely must find it. The "motivation" market has, in some ways, done a great disservice to just how important this is. Motivational speakers may be a dime a dozen now, but that doesn't make finding *your unique motivators* any less important.

Personalize your journey by starting a journal where you list your whys and even your "why nots." What are the reasons why you would *not* work out? I imagine that column will not have very many entries.

Take the time to do the self-care and get to the bottom of your why. Your best friend's why won't cut it. Your spouse's why won't cut it. You have to come up with your own. So, take the time to make it happen.

What's Holding You Back?

If you've read this far and still aren't convinced to get that body moving, then there may be a few other roadblocks standing in your way. We'll discuss a few of them here and why they really aren't the deal breakers you think they are:

The enjoyment factor. If you aren't a gym person or you detest running, then don't do those things. It's pretty simple. Instead, find something you enjoy, because, then, you may actually do it! There are no one-size-fits-all solutions for everyone. What matters is you enjoy it, so you will do it again. Start to think outside the box and come up with alternatives to traditional exercise, and you'll discover a lot of options!

Outside the Box Exercises

- Hula hooping
- Roller skating or rollerblading
- Swimming
- Skipping

- Rebounding on a trampoline
- Ballroom dancing
- Other dancing (line, swing, salsa)
- Goat yoga (yes, yoga with goats)

Never enough time. I feel like we've covered this one thoroughly, but, to reiterate, working out doesn't have to require hours-long sessions that force you to put your daily routine on hold. Make moving a regular part of your family's routine, and everyone will benefit!

Family history and social class. Amazingly (but not surprisingly), your proclivity to exercise is dependent upon whether your family exercised. Social class and race are also tied to movement and obesity. Considerable evidence now exists that people of racial/ethnic minority groups are far more likely to have a sedentary lifestyle compared with their white counterparts.[261] All I can really say to this is that you were born to be you—not to be your parents or your siblings. If you want to feel better, you have to move, and you're the only one who can make that happen for yourself.

Body insecurities. I hear this so much, and it breaks my heart. Listen to me now and listen well. We all have insecurities. I don't have a weight problem and never have (this is probably genetics more than anything else, because I used to eat terribly), but I do *not* like my butt. To me, it looks... droopy. There is also cellulite on my legs. You know what I tell myself whenever I start to think like this?

> "Dani, there are a lot of people in a wheelchair with no legs who would love your cellulite legs."

You don't have to lose a single pound to start appreciating what you've got.

I know that it can be intimidating to be overweight or insecure and walk into a new yoga class or a barre class, or to go to the gym when you're 250, 350, or 400 pounds. The mental stress behind that is a lot to bear.

This reminds me of long ago when I was teaching yoga at my studio in Paducah called True North Yoga. We had a full class, and we were just getting started. The door opened and in walked a woman who was 350 pounds if she was a pound. She didn't cower or look meek or apologize profusely. She just marched right into the middle of that room with her head held high, plopped her mat down, and went into downward dog (in a skirt). I knew she was someone I wanted to be friends with—and 18 years later, we still are.

People who have that kind of cool confidence are more often the exception rather than the rule, but she made an impression on me that I will never forget.

We have not made it easy for the people who really need it. We've not made working out in public really accessible to those who lack confidence in their appearance or physical abilities.

Social media tells you that you're supposed to look a certain way in your yoga pants and work out a certain way. Then you have these ideas when you walk into the studio about how everyone's going to look or how everyone is going to have a friend there except you, and you know you're not going to fit that mold. Thigh gap, little bitty waist, all the things.

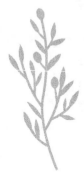

> I don't know who needs to hear this right now, but you really are perfect the way you are.

The whole process just makes us feel inadequate, and it's actually very de-motivating.

The ironic part is you know that girl with the perfect derrière? She looks in the mirror with her clothes off, and she *also* sees something she doesn't like. I guarantee it.

I don't know who needs to hear this right now, but you really are perfect the way you are.

You're not broken. You're perfect. And together, we can turn all of this around for you and get you loving yourself again. But it's going to have to come deep from within.

I saw an ad on Facebook once that said, "Eat what you want and lose weight without exercise! Here's the **final solution** you need to lose weight with zero food restrictions."

What a load of crap!

Who does that ad cater to? Are there still people out there who believe there's a magic bullet to health and weight loss? It's sad that people are so desperate to lose weight and feel better, but they're not desperate enough to change what they eat and start exercising. Well, to that I say this:

You better get busy moving, or you're gonna get busy dying.

I'll add to that statement that you should not eat past satiety, and you should avoid inflammatory foods. *That* is how you lose weight and feel great.

Anything else is just a sleazy marketing gimmick.

I don't think it's ever going to be as easy as, "Finish this chapter and now you're all set and you've got the motivation you need!" Truth be told, it's going to be a daily battle that only *you* are going to be battling. It's you and only you—every dang day.

Just remember that it doesn't have to be fancy. Resolve to move. Put it on your daily to-do list and stop making excuses. Those excuses don't hurt anyone but you.

> **You better get busy moving, or you're gonna get busy dying.**

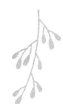

Put movement into your everyday life and feel stronger and better for it!

"You've got to train for it. You've got to eat right. You've got to exercise. Your health account, your bank account, they're the same thing. The more you put in, the more you can take out. Exercise is king and nutrition is queen. Together, you have a kingdom."

JACK LALANNE

wild & well Rx

Dani Williamson, MSN, FNP

R̸ Patient Name: ....

Age: ....   Date: ....

1. Keep it simple, sis or sir! You don't need to spend a lot of money to get fit. Watch old Jack LaLanne videos on YouTube. He will inspire you!

2. Find an exercise buddy to get active and set a date three to four times weekly to move, laugh, and encourage each other.

3. Don't over complicate movement. Get moving during your normal daily routine at work or home.

4. Use pots and pans, laundry detergent, gallons of water, and whatever else you can to lift and build strength.

5. Consider working out in the morning before your day gets started. Make a deal not to eat until you work out. Earn your breakfast!

6. Practice yoga for the many health reasons listed in this chapter. There is a reason it has been around for thousands of years— it works!

7. Start where you are today! No excuses.

8. God made your body perfectly. Thank God for those legs to walk on, those arms to lift with, and those lungs to breathe with and get busy getting stronger.

IN LOVE
- WE TRUST -

"Your gut holds
the key to your
health, and healing
begins within
those walls."

CHAPTER 8

poop well

*"There's three things in this world that you need:
Respect for all kinds of life, a nice bowel movement
on a regular basis, and a navy blazer."*
ROBIN WILLIAMS

Over two thousand years ago, the great physician Hippocrates said, "All disease begins in the gut."

I enthusiastically believe this. I hope that Hippocrates won't mind if I add to it, because I feel that even more significantly, "All *life* begins and ends in the gut."

The gut, otherwise known as your gastrointestinal (GI) tract, along with the liver, pancreas, and gallbladder form the fundamental system of human sustenance, the digestive system. It's a combination of nerves, hormones, microbes, bacteria, blood, and organs that all work together to complete the intricate task of digesting what we consume every day.

I guess we could call it the "command central" for nutrition because every single bite of food we eat, sip of liquid we drink, and pill we take travels through the gut.

If you think digestion begins in the mouth, you might be surprised to learn that digestion begins in the brain. The hypothalamus stimulates appetite, telling us it's time to eat. When we take a bite of food, our brain helps decide how to digest that food—and it will respond with stress or ease, depending on both the health of our systems and our state of mind. Once we respond to the signals put out by our hypothalamus and eat, the intricate process begins.

Oftentimes ignored or at least downplayed by traditional health care providers, the gut is arguably the most discussed and debated and, at the same time, underappreciated system in the body.

I see proof of this sad fact daily, as patient after patient comes to my office begging for help. After just one appointment, I usually learn that at least one of their issues stems from the fact that no medical health professional has ever helped them connect the dots by asking the million-dollar question:

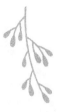

Our health begins from the INSIDE OUT.

What on earth are you eating?

I'm not naïve enough to believe that food sensitivities are the "end all, be all" for our health. However, what I *do* know is that until my patients address their food sensitivities, they find any real healing to be nearly impossible. The reason is simple:

Our health begins from the INSIDE OUT.

So, let's figure out how to bring health back to the gut—that long, connected tube that runs unbroken all the way from the mouth to the anus. The gut's primary functions are:

1. Digestion of food
2. Absorption of nutrients
3. Elimination of waste
4. Immunity

Those first three are not a shocker, but what about that fourth one? Up until a decade or so ago, no one knew the vital and immense role that the gut plays in our health and immunity.

Thanks in large part to the Human Microbiome Project (HMP), a spotlight has been shown on the major influence the gut has on the development and function of the immune system, as well as on gut-brain communications. The HMP was launched in 2007 as a National Institutes of Health (NIH) research initiative. There have been two phases of the initiative so far:[262]

1. The goals of Phase 1 (2007–2014) included exploring the relationship between changes in the microbiome and health/disease by studying several different medical conditions.[263]

2. The goals of Phase 2 (2014–2016) included taking that initial research even further and creating a complete characterization of the human microbiome, with a focus on understanding the presence of microbiota in specific health and disease states.[264]

The research went even deeper, as they looked into how the microbiome changes during pregnancy and influences the *neonatal* microbiome. The project also dove into the role of the microbiome in the occurrence of preterm births, which constitute the second leading cause of neonatal death.[265,266]

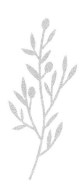

They discovered striking shifts in the microbiome of pre-diabetic patients compared to healthy individuals.

Then they focused on understanding how the gut microbiome changes in those suffering from inflammatory bowel disease (IBD).[267] Researchers found a link between microbiome changes and patients at risk for type 2 diabetes.

They discovered striking shifts in the microbiome of pre-diabetic patients compared to healthy individuals.[268]

The implications of the research are enormous and also are really still in the process of being more fully understood. There is a still a long way to go, but suffice it to say that your gut health is of the utmost importance.

Thanks to the work of those researchers and others, we now know that up to 80 percent of our immune system resides in the gut. That was a game changer for providers (those who choose to stay up to date on new research, that is). Here are a few other takeaways from the studies:[269]

Human Microbiome Project "Gut Punch" Statistics

- About 100 trillion bacteria reside in the gut, and they produce metabolites that have a wide range of health effects.

- An earthworm has more DNA than a human. We are mostly bacteria!

- At least 70 to 80 percent of the body's immune cells are concentrated in the gut.

- There are 100 million neurons located along the gut, which produce various neurotransmitters that regulate mood and satiety.

- Up to 95 percent of the body's total serotonin is located in the gut.

The HMP truly changed the world of gut health by showing that the root cause of chronic lifestyle diseases is inflammation that is linked to adverse changes in our gut bacteria.

Science has shown us that the root of disease is inflammation, and inflammation begins with what goes down the pie hole.

That's a crass way of saying it, but I tend to be blunt when the message is too important to miss.

When the gut is inflamed, you can't absorb the critical nutrients needed to fend off various diseases and conditions. There are multiple conditions associated with poor absorption in the gut. Examples of this include vitamin D and rickets, iron and anemia, B12 and neuropathy, and plenty more.[270]

The struggle to absorb and assimilate starts off gradually and often goes unnoticed for a long time. But eventually, this slowly growing problem leads to a quickly cascading list of health issues.

When I help patients get their gut back on the right track and decrease inflammation, we begin to see their various deficiencies (iron, ferritin, D3, B-12, magnesium RBC, and others) normalize, as if by magic.

It's not magic.

It's the power of a healthy gut!

So, I'll say it again: Your health and your life begin and end in the gut. I'll even take it a step further and say that it begins at birth or before, as the Human Microbiome Project findings showed us.

The time to address digestive health is not when you are *already* suffering from heartburn, bloating, gas, diarrhea, constipation, Celiac Disease, and Crohn's disease. Start addressing it sooner rather than later. I know there's nothing you can do about your own gut at birth, but now you can affect your children's guts and their children's guts.

Research shows that the first 1,000 days of life are critical for setting us up for a lifetime of either feeling good or struggling.[271] We know that the way we entered the world makes a difference in our gut health and our overall health for the rest of our lives. For this reason, we have to consider important factors such as whether a birth was vaginal or a Caesarean section.

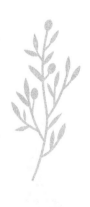

Science has shown us that the root of disease is inflammation, and inflammation begins with what goes down the pie hole.

Many of my patients tell me they struggled with their gut from infancy—and boy, do I believe them! I certainly didn't know about this over two decades ago when I had my kids (and I actually did have two vaginal births), but C-section babies don't get exposed to mom's microbiota in the birth canal and therefore need probiotics! What's fascinating to me is that the research shows that instead of having mom's microbiome, C-section babies have the microbiota found in the operating room, the scrub nurse, and the surgeon.[272]

Isn't that incredible?

Some OB-GYNs today who recognize this and stay up on the latest research allow C-section moms to do vaginal swabs and put their unique microbiome on that sweet baby!

If you are planning to have kids or already had children and had one or more C-sections, don't fret. This is not meant to make you feel guilty. You simply need to be aware that your children's microbiomes may need some supplementation, and you should start following my Wild & Well Gut-Healing Protocol at the end of this chapter with them as soon as possible.

You can make a difference, one little gut at a time.

The Meteoric Rise of Gut Diseases

Sadly, it's obvious from the state of American health and the dramatic increase in gut conditions over the last few decades that precious few of our friends and neighbors are taking care of their lynchpin bodily system. Here are some frightening statistics:[273]

- More than 60 to 70 million Americans suffer on some level with digestive diseases.

- There are more than 95 million Americans with chronic gastrointestinal (GI) disorders.

- Two of the five most prescribed drugs in the country are for digestive disorders.

- Americans spend over $100 billion annually on trying to fix digestive-related problems.

- Colorectal cancer is the second leading cause of cancer deaths behind lung cancer, and it's surprisingly on the rise with the younger population.

These staggering numbers represent patients with an *irritable dowel disease*, or *IBD*, which is an umbrella term used for diseases that cause inflammation in the small intestine and colon. There is a slew of IBDs, but the most common ones include:

- **Irritable Bowel Syndrome.** There are two types—IBS-C (the C stands for constipation) and IBS-D (the D stands for diarrhea). You can switch back and forth between the two or just have one of them. Mine was always IBS-D. IBD sufferers include 13 million people with IBS-C and 16 million with IBS-D.

- **Crohn's Disease.** This condition causes inflammation in the intestinal wall of the small intestine where it joins the large intestine. As of a few years ago, there are as many as three million people suffering from this debilitating disease in our country.[274]

- **Ulcerative Colitis (UC).** UC causes inflammation and ulcers in the lining of the large intestine. The data isn't precise on the number of cases because there are a lot of misdiagnoses in the world of IBDs, but there are at least a million people living with UC in the U.S.

- **Chronic Idiopathic Constipation.** This is diagnosed when a patient shows no signs of physical abnormality, but constipation still occurs. There are an estimated 35 million people living with chronic idiopathic constipation in the U.S.

Want to guess what the word "idiopathic" means? It essentially means doctors don't have a clue why it's happening. My diagnosis from long ago had the word "idiopathic" in there, which is so funny to me now in retrospect, knowing what I know now about how diet and stress affects the gut.

> **Maybe there's a reason why it has the word *idiot* in it— because this ain't rocket science.**

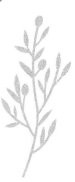

Maybe there's a reason why it has the word *idiot* in it—because this ain't rocket science.

If you can't poop even when you eat fibrous, whole foods, your microbiome needs some serious attention. At the very least, you need to stop consuming all processed foods immediately! Processed foods are inextricably linked to the development of constipation and other IBD symptoms.[275]

Ironically, there isn't an ideal definition for constipation. The definition varies among various studies. All we know for certain is it's considered *idiopathic* and it's more common as you age. Could that be due to reduced gut motility, chronic dehydration, less exercise, inadequate fiber, and more medication?

Yes, to all of the above.

We also know that women are more likely to suffer from constipation during their premenstrual phase each month, and this could be related to fluctuations in female sex hormones.[276] Interestingly, lower economic status sets you up for constipation as well. Lower parental education *and* sexual abuse also contribute to constipation.[277]

Nearly a third of IBD sufferers feel hopeless or depressed due to their condition, and only one in five chronic idiopathic constipation patients feel like they are "in control" of their health.[278]

As many as 81 percent of IBS sufferers work very hard to avoid any place, event, or situation where they don't have easy access to a bathroom.[279] I know this feeling well! I remember declining invites due to the fear that I'd be attacked by a case of surprise diarrhea while there. I've pooped my pants several times in my life, and I'm in no hurry to do it again.

The symptoms of IBD vary a good deal among the various subtypes and include abdominal cramps and/or diffuse pain, fever, weight loss, and diarrhea —sometimes with blood. Compared with adults without IBD, those with IBD are far more likely to have certain chronic health conditions that include:

- Cardiovascular disease
- Respiratory disease
- Cancer
- Arthritis
- Kidney disease
- Liver disease

According to doctors and scientists, there is no cure for IBD.

Patients are told it's genetic and that there is nothing they can do. Doctors will be quick to point out that over 20 percent of people with IBD have another family member with IBD, and families frequently share a similar pattern of disease.[280] That leaves the sufferer feeling stuck for life and resigned to deal with horrible, smelly, painful gut issues until the day they die.

In modern medicine, the goal is to decrease flares and find some normalcy in life through medication. That is done traditionally with prescriptions that include immunosuppressants and steroids to decrease flairs and inflammation.

Sorry, but that's just BS (no pun intended). The goal is not management—it's permanent remission! I'm living proof that this is possible.

I am particularly fascinated with the research that supports this notion because I feel certain I would not have had IBS or lupus had someone addressed my microbiome issues and all the symptoms that go with it as well as my diet in the many years prior to my autoimmune diagnosis.

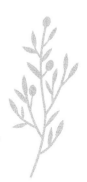

The goal should not be "management" but permanent remission! I'm living proof it's possible.

Allow me to be your cautionary tale, if you aren't already experiencing the debilitating effects of an IBS or a disease like lupus. It was hell on earth, and it was my reality for far too long.

Preventable Suffering is the Worst Kind

I suffered through twenty-four years of bloating, gas, diarrhea, heartburn, itching, and abdominal pain. While I do have a notable ACES score (which we also know is shown to adversely affect our health), I ate very poorly. Even with a garden in our backyard, I opted for processed, packaged, bagged food any chance I got.

I was a Pop Tarts, Cap'n Crunch, Totino's Party Pizza, Betty Crocker icing-loving girl.

I was a Pop Tarts, Cap'n Crunch, Totino's Party Pizza, Betty Crocker icing-loving girl.

I spent years dealing with diarrhea, bloating, and gas before I had my first colonoscopy and IBS diagnosis at age 20. We already talked about my multiple endoscopies and barium enemas earlier in the book, so just let me reiterate that it was no picnic. Multiple gastroenterologists, an overabundance of prescriptions, burping, and nonstop gas. I get chills just thinking about it.

I feel in my gut (literally and figuratively) that my diet and the slew of stopgap treatments and medications to quell my symptoms are what ultimately led to my lupus diagnosis.

My gut was in a constant state of inflammation, and my immune system was "turned on" for so many years. Eventually, those constant triggers "turned on" my autoimmune system, and my body started attacking itself. Still, it took over two decades for a single medical professional to ask me about my diet.

I'm so thankful that I no longer have unpredictable bouts of diarrhea. "Surprise diarrhea" is not a sign of a healthy gut, that's for sure. A healthy gut should not be constipated or experience diarrhea. A healthy gut should not have bloating and gas and gurgling and pain and heartburn every day.

Those gut discomforts are little red flags—or maybe not so little.

We don't pay attention to these kinds of symptoms. We pass them off as "normal" and expected because they are so common. Sorry to burst your bubble, but it's not normal to fart all day, every day. Humans do excrete anywhere from two to four liters of gas a day, but a lot of that happens at night during sleep while the gut is relaxed (maybe your spouse/partner would report that your gut is a little *too* relaxed at night).

Of course, it's also normal to have some gas during the day, but it's not supposed to have the kind of smell that clears the room. That is NOT normal.

When you have a healthy gut, you poop like a dog. Your dog or cat, as a general rule, will go number two shortly after eating a meal. Dogs make it happen neatly and quickly, and then they get excited!

Like our pets, we should also be excited to have a good poop! It's a sign that you are eating whole, fibrous foods and that your gut is healthy.

Speaking of good poop, do you know what a good poop is supposed to look like?

Water makes up about 75 percent of your stool. The rest is a stinky combination of fiber, dead and live bacteria, other cells, and mucus. Soluble fiber found in foods like beans and nuts is broken down during digestion and forms a gel-like substance that becomes part of your fecal matter.

Foods packed with insoluble fiber, such as corn, oat bran, and carrots, are more difficult for your body to digest, which explains why they may emerge in your stool looking relatively unchanged. I tell patients if they aren't sure how fast or slow their transit time is, they just need to eat some corn on the cob (organic, non-GMO, heirloom) and see how long it takes to notice the kernels in their stool. It's a little gross, but it's also a simple experiment. The rule of thumb is:

What you eat today should be gone by tomorrow.

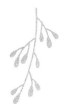

What you eat today should be gone by tomorrow.

Do you look at your poop? When I ask my patients what their poop looks like, most people don't want any part of that. If that sounds like you, then you are going to have to start looking in that toilet bowl—because these are questions you need to know the answers to!

- Is there any visible food?
- Is it cracked or smooth?
- Is it skinny like a noodle or fat?
- Is it clay colored or darker?
- Does it float or sink?
- It is slimy?

People don't like to look and, because of that, they are missing key elements about their health. A light-colored poop often indicates a gallbladder issue. Slimy poop and floaters are also not good. Floating is a sign of too much fat in your diet and malabsorption in the gut. Those are just a few of the many things your poop can tell you.

Funny but True:

The really good poopers of the world who are interested in seeing what comes out of them can't stand automatic flushers in a bathroom. Before they stand up, the poop is down the drain—and that irritates the crap out of them (pun definitely intended).

the bristol
stool chart

type 1	**SEVERE CONSTIPATION** *Separate hard lumps, like nuts*
type 2	**MILD CONSTIPATION** *Lumpy and sausage like*
type 3	**NORMAL** *Sausage shape with surface cracks*
type 4	**NORMAL** *Like a smooth, soft sausage or snake*
type 5	**LACKING FIBER** *Soft blobs with clear-cut edges*
type 6	**MILD DIARRHEA** *Mushy consistency with ragged edges*
type 7	**SEVERE DIARRHEA** *Liquid consistency with no solid pieces*

I've been using the *Bristol Stool Chart* for years to help my patients become poop detectives. I've even got a giant one up on the wall in my office for every single patient to look at and discuss.

As you can see in the chart on the previous page, there are seven basic types of poo.

The ideal result is to have a Type 4 on the Bristol Stool Chart, two to three times daily.

Patients report to me regularly that their previous doctor told them it's okay to poop just two to three times a week. That is *not* okay under any circumstances! If you are not pooping at least once a day, you need to take immediate steps to fix that.

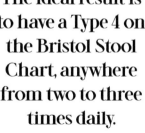

The ideal result is to have a Type 4 on the Bristol Stool Chart, anywhere from two to three times daily.

Part of the reason we don't evacuate like we should is that humans were designed to squat while we poop.

Squatting helps open all the muscles down there and get that waste out of your body! One tool that has helped me greatly and that I recommend to everyone is a Squatty Potty (or something similar upon which to rest your feet). This is important because when you sit with your legs down, your sphincter muscles *contract*, but when you squat, those muscles *relax*.

I love the Squatty Potty brand because it tucks under the toilet nicely, but you can put your feet up on anything: the trash can, a block, your dog, a child who won't leave the bathroom.

If you can't relate to the excitement your dog feels after a poop, then there could be many factors at play. One of the most adverse conditions is called *intestinal permeability*, more commonly known as *leaky gut*. It's a condition that you need to know more about. So, we'll spend the next few sections teaching you about the ecosystem that governs your intestines, and you'll get a brief lesson on what leaky gut is and how it's hurting you.

I didn't learn about leaky gut in nurse practitioner school. I can't speak to nursing school today, but I know that I never even heard the terms "leaky gut" or "intestinal permeability" uttered one time. Isn't that *sad*? There's really no other word for it. It's sad that the majority of traditional medical professionals do not learn about this critical topic.

How do intelligent people (doctors are some of the smartest people around) reconcile in their heads that diet and the health of the gut have nothing to do with overall health?

I can't speak for other practitioners. All I know is that patients tell me every day that they hear things from gastroenterologist and other gut specialists like, "If you want to take a probiotic, you can. There's some research on it, but it's not conclusive," and that's about as deep as they'll dive into the microbiome.

Medical schools don't teach true "healthcare" education. It's all about what to do once you're already sick. *It's sickcare.* A symptoms-based approach is what rules modern medicine. If I had found a functional medicine practitioner all those years ago, would my life have turned out differently? I am certain of it! However, you don't get do-overs. All you can do is make better choices today so that you can have a healthier tomorrow.

Thank God I'm far down the road toward healing. Yes, I'm still a work in progress. I still have food sensitivities and bouts of gas, but I am so much better than I ever was. I am thankful to know the truth and won't ever go back to eating like I once did.

As much as I love them, my mouth tasted its last Pop Tart many years ago.

I know how critical the gut is to our health! In fact, I'm such a big believer in the gut being the key to it all that I got a personalized license plate to tell the world.

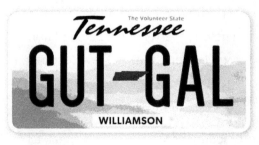

So, if you're ever driving around Franklin, Tennessee and see a car with a customized **"GUT GAL"** license plate, go ahead and give me a beep, beep and a wave.

When Your Ecosystem Springs a Leak

The relationship between the *gut microbiota* and human health and immunity is being increasingly recognized. Thanks to the groundbreaking work conducted through the Human Microbiome Project (HMP), it is now well established that a healthy gut flora is largely responsible for the overall health of its host.

There are three to ten times more microorganisms living inside the microbiome than there are human cells in the whole body!

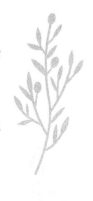

Yep, we're the hosts, or, more precisely, our gut is the host. The gut is the home to over 100 trillion microorganisms, collectively known as the *gut microbiota* that make up the microbiome. We're talking about the enormous collection of foreign organisms that reside inside our bodies—and particularly within our GI tract—that serve to create a mini-ecosystem inside us.

There are three to ten times more microorganisms living inside the microbiome than there are human cells in the whole body!

These microbes have the power to affect just about every aspect of our health—from metabolism and weight to our immunity and moods.[281]

Researchers have even found that we emit our own distinct, personal "microbial cloud." We are constantly interacting with microbes that other people have left behind on chairs, in the air, and on every surface we touch. Add these interactions to the ones we have with microbes that pets leave, those that blow off leaves and soil, and those in food and water, and that's a recipe for a limitless amount of microbial combinations.

I like to imagine it like we're all Pigpen from the *Peanuts* cartoon, walking around with a cloud of microbes following behind us everywhere we go.

Those limitless combinations make every individual's microbiome truly unique. Two people who are both considered to be "healthy" can have vastly different populations of microbiota living inside their bodies and on their skin.[282]

Increasing bodies of research are making it clear that humans have developed alongside these complex microbial interactions, and that we now depend on them for our very wellbeing.[283]

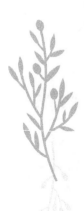

> **Many researchers now believe that a diverse population of microorganisms is perhaps the biggest key to remaining disease-free.**

Many researchers now believe that a diverse population of microorganisms is perhaps the biggest key to remaining disease-free.

We have this special, symbiotic relationship with the trillions of microbes that live inside our bodies, especially inside our guts. *Symbiosis* refers to a mutually beneficial relationship between two organisms. In other words, we help these organisms survive, and in turn, they help regulate many of our bodily functions.

And the goal, as is the case in any ecosystem, is to live in harmony (aka homeostasis).

Dysbiosis is when we have more bad bacteria than good bacteria. Our immune system is responsible for two things: allowing the good bacteria to live and thrive and attacking the bad bacteria. But when the gut is impaired in some way, it doesn't work like that.

One example of this in action is when researchers showed that type 2 diabetes patients have an overabundance of bad bacteria, or a constant state of *dysbiosis*, in their guts.[284] The same link is now being made to dysbiosis and hypertension, depression, Alzheimer's disease, and more.[285]

Explains a lot, doesn't it?

The downfall of the gut and what makes us so suspectable to this state of dysbiosis can often be linked to a condition known as intestinal permeability, or *leaky gut*.

The GI barrier is an intricate and selective wall that controls and permits the absorption of nutrients into the bloodstream while keeping out harmful substances. When you are healthy, the gut is tightly regulated, allowing only important nutrients to pass through, and protects you from harmful substances such as toxins, undigested food, and pathogens.

leaky gut

The gastrointestinal (GI) barrier is an intricate and selective wall that controls and permits the absorption of nutrients into the bloodstream while keeping out substances that are harmful. When you are healthy, the gut is tightly regulated, allowing only important nutrients to pass through, and protecting you from harmful substances such as toxins, undigested food, and pathogens. Since the gut is constantly exposed to inflammatory foods, medicines, and chemicals, the GI tract must work feverishly to defend itself from attack. If allowed entry into the body, the harmful substances can leak into your bloodstream and cause inflammation. The constant exposure to foreign substances can cause the walls of the intestines to become vulnerable to deterioration and permeability, and this is the condition commonly referred to as leaky gut syndrome.

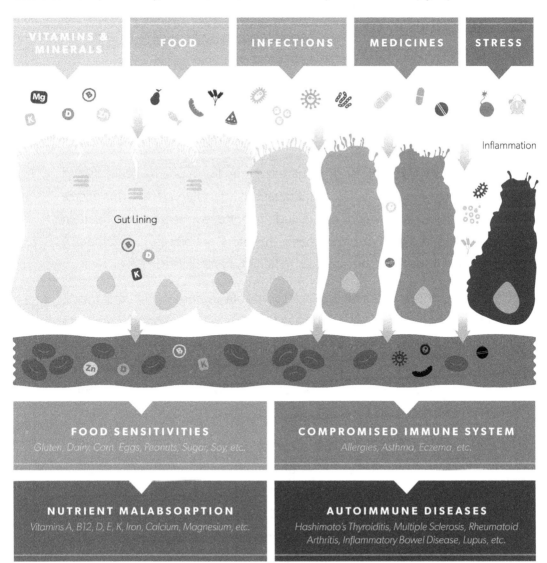

VITAMINS & MINERALS

FOOD

INFECTIONS

MEDICINES

STRESS

Inflammation

Healthy

Gut Lining

Unhealthy

FOOD SENSITIVITIES
Gluten, Dairy, Corn, Eggs, Peanuts, Sugar, Soy, etc.

COMPROMISED IMMUNE SYSTEM
Allergies, Asthma, Eczema, etc.

NUTRIENT MALABSORPTION
Vitamins A, B12, D, E, K, Iron, Calcium, Magnesium, etc.

AUTOIMMUNE DISEASES
Hashimoto's Thyroiditis, Multiple Sclerosis, Rheumatoid Arthritis, Inflammatory Bowel Disease, Lupus, etc.

Since the gut is constantly exposed to inflammatory foods, medicines, and chemicals, the GI tract must work feverishly to defend itself from attack. If allowed entry into the body, the harmful substances can leak into your bloodstream and cause inflammation.

The constant exposure to foreign substances can cause the walls of the intestines to become vulnerable to deterioration and permeability, and this is what results in leaky gut syndrome.

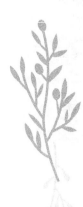

Having leaky gut is like having the gates broken from your intestines to your blood stream, so that many harmful particles that should never have been able to enter can now get through.

Having leaky gut is like having the gates broken from your intestines to your blood stream, so that many harmful particles that should never have been able to enter can now get through.

When this happens, it causes inflammation throughout your body, leading to a variety of symptoms, ailments, and diseases.

There is a long list of pharmaceuticals and medications that damage the gut microbiome and lead to leaky gut that include hypertensive medications, certain antidepressants, NSAIDS, proton pump inhibitors, antibiotics, chemotherapy agents, and more that can all be toxic to healthy bacteria.

Of course, not all medications are avoidable in certain circumstances. You can't beat yourself up if you have to take a prescription, but you also have to recognize that you're depleting something in your gut by taking it, and, therefore, the gut will need assistance getting balanced again. For example, if you are taking TUMS for heartburn, it depletes zinc in your body. So, you need to supplement with zinc or eat more zinc-rich foods to make up for this.

I know it can be daunting to ask, "But won't this affect my gut?" and other probing questions when you are at the doctor's office. So many people feel intimidated to ask their doctors the "why" behind what they are experiencing or even what they can expect from a medication. Instead, they just do what they are told and take the medicine. After all:

"Who are *you* to question the experts?"

"Did *you* go to medical school?"

I've even had patients tell me their provider said to them, "Oh, yeah? So, where's your medical degree?"

It's hubris like that it is destroying the trust that once existed between doctors and their patients. Medical professionals are human, too, and we are prone to the same biases and also to the human tendency to be averse to change. The bottom line is this:

Doctors are *down* on things they're not *up* on. It's as simple as that. So, here is what I suggest:

The next time you are at the doctor's office, ask them what they thought about the Human Microbiome Project findings. It will be interesting to hear what they say. If you find a doctor who acknowledges the critical link between the microbiome and overall health, you may just be able to start to get the answers you need to experience inside-out healing.

Join Me on Facebook!

I encourage you to go to Facebook and join my private group aptly named **"Inside Out—Healing From Within."** Thousands of members help each other daily answer health questions and provide a community of support!

The Gut-Brain Connection

Gut health is now being linked to neurological issues including depression, Alzheimer's, and dementia—and there's a reason for that. Every system in our body is inextricably linked to the others. However, this is *especially* true in the case of the gut and nervous system.

Digestive processes provide the building blocks for many functions of the nervous system. This includes fueling the brain and producing vital neuro-transmitters such as serotonin and dopamine.[286]

Newer research points to the undeniable fact that not only is there a *gut-immune* connection, but there is also a *gut-brain* connection, and that the health of this connection is essential for maintaining homeostasis within the central nervous system.

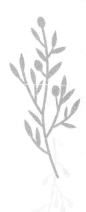

Forward-thinking researchers describe the relationship between the digestive system and nervous system as a two-way street.

In fact, there is now expanding evidence suggesting that organisms within the gut play a role in early neural programming.

Forward-thinking researchers describe the relationship between the digestive system and nervous system as a two-way street.

Digestion supplies the nervous system with necessary fuel and alerts the brain of potential threats, and, in return, the nervous system controls aspects of the digestive tract.

The brain is also in charge of controlling muscles in the GI tract, and it controls signals that affect elimination and appetite regulation.

Throughout the day, the digestive system picks up "signals" from the body and sends sensory information back to the brain about the body's overall state of health and emotional wellbeing. This is one reason why people may say that they have a "gut feeling" about something.

When you are nervous, you might get an upset stomach because of the gut-brain connection. This feeling is commonly referred to as "butterflies in the stomach," which often happens before a big presentation, test, or performance.

More proof of the gut-brain connection is the assertion by scientists that **migraine headaches generally stem from digestive malfunction.** Here's how they explain it:

The gut has its own nervous system—sometimes called the *second brain*—and when the gut is functioning at optimal levels, it produces adequate serotonin. That is significant because migraines involve "excitable neurons" that can be calmed by serotonin. When the digestive system is not properly functioning, it is not capable of producing the amounts of serotonin needed to sufficiently quell these neurons, and they become inflamed, causing the pain associated with migraines.[287]

Your head may ache when you have a migraine, but it may be really your gut that's hurting!

A recent study has also shown a link between migraines and food allergies (this is certainly no surprise to me!). In a study of five hundred migraine patients, more than 60 percent of them tested positive for allergies to dairy, 50 percent had sensitivities to wheat and grain, and 35 percent displayed allergies to eggs.[288]

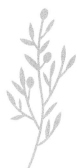

> **Your head may ache when you have a migraine, but it may be really your gut that's hurting!**

Get tested for food allergies/sensitivities ASAP if you suffer from regular headaches or migraines! There *is* a reason for your pain—you just haven't dug long or far enough yet to find the root. I tell patients that when we heal their gut, we also begin to heal the nervous system. I have the privilege of frequently watching my patients decrease their anxiety and depression medications as we heal their guts.

You may need Prozac, but it's not because of a Prozac deficiency. Find the root and remove the need to cover up the symptoms.

Are you going to be able to stop all of your medications right now or never take another pill again? If you have a health condition that requires medication, likely not (and don't make any changes to what you take without talking with a doctor first).

> **You may need Prozac, but it's not because of a Prozac deficiency. Find the root and remove the need to cover up the symptoms.**

Just know that you *can* heal your gut, even if you take prescriptions. Antibiotics, in particular, are damaging to the gut. According to the CDC, of the hundreds of millions of prescriptions that are written for antibiotics each year, as many as 30 percent of them are unnecessary.[289]

Yikes.

Ultimately, it's not your doctor's responsibility to keep you healthy. I know this is contradictory to what we've been told or how we see things—but it's true. **You alone are responsible for your health.** If you have to take an antibiotic or other drug, do what you have to do, but then take responsibility for your own health and learn to how to restore your gut flora to healthy, symbiotic levels afterwards. Then take proactive steps (like my Wild & Well Gut-Healing Protocol at the end of this chapter) to avoid leaky gut and keep your internal ecosystem happy and thriving.

Supplements that Support the Gut

Poor gut health is tied to nearly every disease in some way, because the gut is where much of the immune system lives and where inflammation often begins. Improving your diet and getting a food sensitivity test, drinking lots of clean water, lowering stress, and exercising regularly are among the best ways to support the body's microbiome and attain an optimal level of health. However, there are also a few key supplements that I recommend. We'll start with the one that I advocate most often.

1. PROBIOTICS

If there is one supplement that I recommend absolutely everyone take, from kids to adults, it's probiotics. In a perfect world, you should be getting sufficient amounts of both probiotics and prebiotics (that act as a source of food for your gut bacteria) in food.

Thanks to modern eating habits, however, that is just not going to happen for most people.

Digestive experts agree that the balance of gut flora should be approximately 85 percent good bacteria and 15 percent bad bacteria. If this ratio gets out of balance, you develop *dysbiosis*, which means there's an imbalance of too much of a certain type of fungus, yeast, or bacteria that affects the body in a negative way.

Probiotics are the "good bugs." They compete for space with bad bacteria, promote the release of natural antibodies in the digestive tract, and can even attack unhealthy bacteria. Your good gut bacteria are also responsible for producing vitamin B12, butyrate, and vitamin K2 as well as stimulating the secretion of immunoglobulin A (also known as IgA) and regulatory T-cells.

Through stimulation of bacterial growth and fermentation, probiotics promote healthy bowel habits and can also help loosen up your bowels and help you poop more easily (with the goal of getting you to a Type 4 on the Bristol Stool Chart at least twice a day).[290] By adding more probiotic foods into your diet and taking a good probiotic supplement, you may experience the following:

- Stronger immune system

- Healing from leaky gut and IBD

- Improved digestion

- Increased energy from production of vitamin B12

- Better breath (probiotics help destroy *Candida*)

- Healthier skin (probiotics naturally treat eczema and psoriasis)

- Reduced incidences and/or severity of illness

- Weight loss

Not all probiotics are created equally, and there are A LOT of utterly useless ones out there.

With all of the press that probiotics have been receiving for the past several years, even mainstream food manufacturers have jumped into the action. Your multivitamin, your smoothie, and even your pizza may now claim to "contain probiotics." The reason is simple—it's big business. The probiotic food market has reached over $45 billion and climbing.

The best way to take in probiotics is through natural food sources such as sour, fermented, and probiotic-rich foods (kimchi, kefir, sauerkraut, apple cider vinegar, etc.). A close second is a high-quality probiotic supplement.

Watch my videos about probiotics on YouTube at Dani Williamson Wellness. We have several, and you will learn so much! There are four specific things you want to consider when buying a probiotic supplement:

1. **Brand quality**—Look for brands that are reputable. My personal favorites are Theralac, Mega Spore, Metagenics, and Orthomolecular.

2. **High CFU count**—Purchase a probiotic brand that has a higher number of probiotics, from 15 billion to 100 billion.

3. **Strain diversity**—Search for a probiotic supplement that has multiple strains and strands (the goal is gut diversity).

4. **Survivability**—Look for strains such as *Bacillus coagulans*, *Saccharomyces boulardii*, *Bacillus subtilis*, *Lactobacillus rhamnosus*, and other cultures or formulas that ensure probiotics make it to the gut and are able to colonize.

Ultimately, we want a probiotic that will protect its host (me and you) from the damaging act of eating food! There is a little known but surprisingly common condition called **metabolic endotoxemia**, and it's associated with some scary stuff such as metabolic disorders, type 2 diabetes, obesity, heart disease, and autoimmunity. Here is what you need to know about it...

Lipopolysaccharides (LPSs) are endotoxins found on the outside of some of our gut bacteria. About five hours after we eat, those toxins are released into the gut. In healthy people, the LPSs stay inside the gut wall and don't cause any problems. However, if you have a leaky gut, the compromised gut wall lets LPSs through into the bloodstream.

An increased level of LPSs/endotoxins in the blood results in metabolic endotoxemia, and it causes long-term, slow-burning, chronic inflammation. The condition has been linked to high-fat diets (or more accurately, high junk diets), so make sure your fats are clean and from organic (if possible), whole-food sources.[291]

Probiotics Pro-Tip

Don't buy a probiotics supplement that requires refrigeration. If it can't even survive room temperature, how is it going to survive the perilous voyage to your intestines? You need one that is shelf-stable and has patented delivery system with a capsule that will survive the journey through the gut. If you have a refrigerated one, make sure the capsule is one that survives the journey.

One recent review showed that both probiotics and prebiotics help prevent LPSs from leaking out into the bloodstream in the first place, so find a good supplement and start healing and preventing inflammation.[292]

2. IMMUNOGLOBULINS

In the previous section, I mentioned that probiotics stimulate the secretion of immunoglobulins. So, in theory, a healthy body produces enough of the antibodies known as immunoglobulins (IgGs) on its own.

There are actually five types of immunoglobulins: IgA, IgD, IgE, IgG, and IgM. These immune-fighting antibodies help heal and protect the gut lining. The body is supposed to make them in response to foreign substances, or antigens, such as bacteria, viruses, fungi, animal dander, and even cancer cells.

The immunoglobulins attach to the foreign substances, signaling to the immune system to go into "search and destroy" mode. I suppose you could say they act like Pac-Man, going around and gobbling up all the bad stuff. When immunoglobulins bind to an antigen, this act triggers inflammation as well as an immune response to clean up the damage.

A little inflammation is not bad if there is an important job to be done. However, if your immunoglobulins are constantly fighting harmful toxins, it leads to a state of chronic inflammation and potentially leaky gut.

The best way to avoid this is to support the immune system by more effectively attacking invading toxins and, at the same time, rebuilding the gut barrier. An IgG-based supplement will help with something called *passive immunity*. A high-quality IgG supplement delivers IgG directly to your gut and helps bind more toxins, which can calm inflammation caused

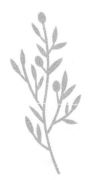

Oral IgG supplements have shown tremendous results in patients with IBD.

by those toxins long enough for your gut to begin to heal. My personal favorite is from Microbiome Labs. It's a powdered IgG drink sourced from bovine and is incredible at healing the gut lining and decreasing inflammation. My son swears it healed his gut when he got sick in Bangkok a few years ago.

Oral IgG supplements have shown tremendous results in patients with IBD.

For example, in one human trial, after just eight weeks of using a serum-derived bovine immunoglobulin supplement, the subjects' loose bowel movements reduced by 50 percent![293]

I use a powder form for most of my patients and a new oral form with spore-based probiotics as well. Look for one that is a serum-derived bovine immunoglobulin supplement, and steer clear of the many copycat products that use colostrum (dairy milk) as their IgG source.

3. DIGESTIVE ENZYMES

The phrase "you are what you eat" is a bit of a misconception. Truth be told, you are what you *digest*—and digestive enzymes are key to both better digestion and nutrient absorption.

The role of digestive enzymes is primarily to act as catalysts in speeding up specific, life-preserving chemical reactions in the body. Essentially, they help break down larger molecules into more easily absorbed particles that the body can use to survive and thrive.

In a perfect world, the body makes enough enzymes to support healthy digestion. However, thanks to the way most people eat (the SAD diet), chemicals in our food, toxins in our environments, and other modern issues, supplementation is often necessary. There are several great reasons to take a digestive enzyme supplement:

- Helps heal leaky gut by taking stress off the GI tract.

- Assists the body in breaking down difficult-to-digest substances.

- Improves symptoms of acid reflux and IBD.

- Enhances nutrition absorption and prevents nutritional deficiency.

- Counteracts senzyme inhibitors naturally in foods such as peanuts, wheat, eggs, nuts, seeds, beans, and potatoes.

Digestive enzyme products are derived from three sources: 1) Fruit-sourced, usually pineapple- or papaya-based; 2) Animal-sourced, including pancreatin sourced from ox or hog; and 3) Plant-sourced, from probiotics, yeast, and fungi. Look for a "full-spectrum" enzyme blend for general digestive improvement. As a bonus, you can opt for a blend with herbs such as peppermint and ginger that also. support digestion.

4. L-GLUTAMINE

L-glutamine is the most plentiful amino acid in the body. It's also helpful because it aids in decreasing inflammation and healing leaky gut. The tissues in the intestine use L-glutamine as a fuel source to function at their best. L-glutamine is also thought to help maintain proper barriers within the intestine, which is why it's known to be a great supplement for leaky gut sufferers. Dr. Cheryl Burdette of Precision Point Diagnostics Lab (our food sensitivity testing source) calls L-glutamine "spackling for the gut." It literally helps patch up a leaky gut.

Studies suggest that some cases of IBD may occur due to an L-glutamine deficiency. Researchers have reported that patients who increase their intake of L-glutamine may notice a reduction or disappearance of their symptoms due to the fact that the L-glutamine works to restore and protect the mucous membrane of the gut.[294]

The beauty of L-glutamine for many of my patients is that it also helps with carb, sugar, and alcohol cravings. I even use it for anxiety patients, as it has a calming effect on the nervous system.

5. LICORICE ROOT

Licorice root is an adaptogenic herb with four key compounds: flavonoids, coumarins, triterpenoids, and stilbenoids. The triterpenoid glycyrrhizin is what gives licorice root its anti-inflammatory, laxative, and expectorant properties. For healthy adults, glycyrrhizin can be consumed for its many health benefits, including aiding gut health.

A study published in Evidence-based Complementary and Alternative Medicine evaluated the efficacy of an extract of glycyrrhizin glabra against "functional dyspepsia," a blanket term that includes heartburn, nausea, indigestion, and stomach pain. Researchers found that the extract showed a significant decrease in total symptom scores after fifteen and thirty days of treatment. The extract was also found to be safe and well tolerated by all patients.[295] Other benefits of licorice root include:

- Relieves heartburn and acid reflux

- Fights nausea and stomach pain

- Improves leaky gut

- Helps heal stomach ulcers and canker sores

- Boosts the immune system

The recommended dose for licorice root extract is a maximum of six grams a day for a 130-pound person. Be sure to choose deglycyrrhizinated (DGL) licorice because it has the substantial parts of glycyrrhizin removed. This dosage limits the amount of glycyrrhizin being consumed (the reason this is important is because with excessive use, glycyrrhizin could create side effects such as increased blood pressure, reduced potassium levels, edema, and other issues).

There are standardized supplements available without this compound, making the product generally safer for widespread sales. The one I use in my office is called MegaGuard, and it's phenomenal for addressing both *H. pylori* and heartburn. Licorice extract should not be taken for more than four weeks at a time. DGL licorice can be taken longer, but a break between uses is still recommended.

6. PREBIOTICS

I'm a big fan of *prebiotics*, which are indigestible fiber foods that help prepare the gut for the probiotics to do their job. Our gut microbiome needs "fuel" to keep functioning optimally. Prebiotics are designed to do just that. As a bonus, prebiotics can help aid in:

- Weight loss.

- Stronger immune system.

- Improved digestion and regular bowel movements.

- Better heart health and lower cholesterol.

- Enhanced oral health.

- Elevated energy and boosted mood.

Prebiotics are resistant to human digestion, which means they pass through the small intestine into the large intestine, where they are then broken down by the good bugs and converted into health-promoting substances such as short-chain fatty acids (SCFAs). The best possible way to take in prebiotics is through food. Three of the top sources in our diet are:

1. Resistant oligosaccharides—found in glutinous foods, onion, and garlic.

2. Resistant starch—found in foods such as green bananas, oats, and cooked and cooled rice, pasta, and potatoes.

3. Phytonutrients—found in many fruits, vegetables, whole grains, nuts, and legumes.

Dr. Tom O'Bryan is a recognized world expert on gluten and its impact on health. He suggests that one great (and delicious) way to take in more prebiotics is to make organic stewed apples. You simply cook them until they're soft and shimmery. Dr. O'Bryan explains that this releases *pectin*—a soluble fiber that provides fuel for our beneficial gut bacteria.

Eat more prebiotic-rich foods to help build diversity, or you can also choose to take a supplement. Like always, quality matters. Be sure to look for one that has a diversity of both fructo-oligosaccharides (FOS) and galacto-oligosaccharides (GOS). You need both as well as gum arabic. It also needs to be organic and additive-free. Finally, make sure your supplement is manufactured in cGMP-certified facilities and quality tested after production.

7. PEPPERMINT

Peppermint is a hybrid species of spearmint and water mint. Peppermint may be the most versatile essential oil in the world. There are few body, health, and mind issues that it cannot help. This is especially true for your gut.

The health benefits and uses of peppermint oil have been documented back before the days of Jesus. Peppermint oil is recommended for its anti-nausea benefits and soothing effects on the gastric lining and colon because of its ability to reduce muscle spasms. Some of the other potential benefits of peppermint oil include:

- Soothes gut distress
- Freshens breath
- Relieves headaches
- Improves mental focus
- Boosts energy
- Helps clear the respiratory tract
- Releases tight muscles
- Serves as a natural alternative to NSAIDs taken for pain

Peppermint oil taken internally in capsule form has been proven to be effective at naturally treating IBS. One study found a 50-percent reduction in IBS symptoms with 75 percent of patients who used it.[296]

Add a drop of food-grade, organically sourced peppermint oil to your water bottle, rub a few drops behind your ears, or diffuse it to help reduce nausea and aid with digestive issues. It can also be beneficial as a part of your diet.

A few more of my favorite gut-supporting supplements that you may consider are:

* **Artichoke leaf.** Artichoke leaf can help improve digestive function, lower cholesterol levels, and provide liver protection. After two months of using an artichoke leaf extract, 208 patients with IBS reported a 26-percent reduction in IBS symptoms.[297]

* **Apple cider vinegar.** Raw apple cider vinegar (ACV) may help improve digestion, calm your skin, and aid with nutrient absorption. Despite the fact that ACV itself is acidic, it actually helps promote an alkaline environment in your body, boost metabolism, and support the repair of your gut lining.[298]

* **Aloe vera.** Aloe vera provides a cooling, soothing relief from digestive distress. It contains prebiotic compounds that help feed healthy probiotics, and it's also helpful for reducing the symptoms of acid reflux.

When it comes to the duration for taking supplements, I recommend taking a new supplement for three months and then assessing how effective it is. I also recommend changing probiotic brands every three months or so to keep the diversity of the strains in your microbiome as high as possible.

Dani's Wild & Well Gut-Healing Protocol

I hope by now you are incredibly clear on one thing: What you eat determines how you feel, and it also determines the health of your gut. When it comes to maintaining a healthy gut and avoiding intestinal permeability, you should be willing to stop at nothing to heal your gut! Here are my steps for achieving a healthy gut and, therefore, a healthier life:

1. GET TESTED FOR FOOD SENSITIVITIES.

The first step in my Wild & Well Gut-Healing Protocol is always to get tested for food sensitivities. I'm a big believer in healing through elimination.

You take away things that are adversely affecting you rather than add in a supplement or prescription to mask symptoms.

The food sensitivity tests we do in my office checks a total of 88 foods. You need to know which foods your body likes, and which ones are causing inflammation. This is a critical and essential first step in healing your gut.

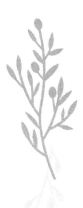

> **You take away things that are adversely affecting you rather than add in a supplement or prescription to mask symptoms.**

Cutting out the top seven—gluten, dairy, soy, corn, sugar, eggs, and peanuts—is key, but many of my patients react to other foods, and some of those foods are a real shock to them. I've seen patients have sensitivities to beef, avocados, blueberries, and a number of normally healthy spices and herbs. It's fascinating how a super food may be "super" for some people, but not for *you*!

Are you thinking to yourself, "There's no way an avocado could be doing anyone any harm!" I know—it's hard to believe. But for my patients who, through testing, are shown to have an avocado sensitivity, the proof is in the pudding. When they stop eating avocados, their inflammation cools and their gut health improves.

If you can't afford to get tested right now, cut out the Sinister Seven first and see how you feel. Then, I recommend you add in a great probiotic and a digestive enzyme at a minimum.

2. EAT THE WILD & WELL WAY.

If you need a refresher, it's time to go back to Chapter Five and re-read the best way to eat for healing and total body restoration. Once you remove the

Sinister Seven, there are still so many delicious foods to eat that won't cause inflammation and lead to gut issues.

Taste the rainbow with every meal by eating a wide variety of fruits and veggies, eat clean meat, drink *lots* of water, and consume ancient grains from time to time (as long as you don't have a sensitivity to them).

It's really not hard to eat well. You are just not in the habit. So, get in the habit by making your meals at home using whole-food ingredients and start feeling good after meals again!

3. EAT FERMENTED FOODS AND SUPPLEMENT WITH PROBIOTICS.

In addition to taking a high-quality probiotic, it's a good idea to include foods in your diet that contain lots of the "good bugs" that help your gut thrive. Eating fermented foods helps to increase gut diversity.

Fermented foods are one of the best things we know traditionally that are going to help the good bacteria in your gut thrive (if you have histamine issues, you will want to limit fermented foods). They go a long way toward protecting you and your immune system. Aim to eat a forkful of fermented veggies twice a day and see how much better you start to feel. The best fermented foods to supplement your diet include:

1. Yogurt (made from coconuts or goat's milk)

2. Apple cider vinegar

3. Kombucha (low in sugar)

4. Kimchi

5. Sauerkraut

6. Kefir

7. Miso

8. Tempeh

As I mentioned before, in a perfect world, you would eat all the probiotics you need, and you wouldn't have to take a supplement. If you want to aim for that, I say go for it!

4. RESTORE THE GUT AFTER ANTIBIOTIC USE.

A few decades ago, most people never thought twice about taking a round of antibiotics for anything, even if a virus was the cause of an illness (and therefore not affected by an antibiotic). Today we know that the overuse of antibiotics has caused some significant issues.

Antibiotics clean the body of dangerous germs, but they also eliminate good bacteria from the gut, which means they can lower immune function and raise the risk for future infections, allergies, and diseases.

Antibiotics have the power to save lives when they are truly needed, but they are often over-prescribed and misunderstood. To make matters worse, according to research published in *Frontiers in Microbiology*, the human microbiome is overly exposed to antibiotics due not only to their medical use, but also to their utilization in farm animals and crops.[299]

Our food supply is so messed up!

Our food supply is so messed up!

Researchers found that microbiome composition can be rapidly altered by exposure to antibiotics, with potential immediate detrimental effects on health.[300] Microbiome alterations induced by antibiotics can also indirectly affect health in the long-term. Before using antibiotics, just make sure it's something you *really* need.

If you do need one, take steps to restore gut flora. Here are some ways to help your gut after antibiotics:

* The general rule of thumb is to do at least one month of probiotic treatment for every week that you are on antibiotics. Of course, I say the longer, the better.

* If you have been on antibiotics for an extended period, you may have a severe erosion of the glycocalyx that normally coats the intestines. This will likely result in a notable reduction in secretory IgA production. In this case, you'll need to find a probiotic strain that includes *Saccharomyces boulardii*, an antibiotic-resistant, probiotic yeast originally isolated from lychee fruit in Indochina.

- Other plant-based medicines such as oregano oil, tea tree oil, and pau d'arco extract can further help rid the GI tract of pathogenic yeast caused by antibiotic use.

- Eats lots of both probiotic and prebiotic foods daily.

- Butyrate is another key player in gut bacteria restoration. It's a natural substance made in the intestine, and antibiotics may reduce production. In that case, consider supplementation.

5. EXERCISE AND BE ACTIVE EVERY SINGLE DAY.

We are about to talk about exercise and movement a lot more in the next chapter, so for now, I'll just point out that exercise is a natural stress reliever that can help lower inflammation, balance hormones, and strengthen the immune system.[301] Moving the body also helps to keep food moving through the digestive system. Exercise increases blood flow to the organs and engages muscles in the GI tract.

Research conducted at the University of California at Irvine found that moderate exercise can benefit patients with IBD and liver disease. Researchers proved that physical exercise could improve gastric emptying and lower the relative risk of colon cancer. Severe, exhaustive exercise, however, inhibited gastric emptying and interfered with gastrointestinal absorption.[302]

So, get moving but choose movements that bring healing to your body rather than more stress on the gut. For more on exercise, see Chapter Eight.

6. ACTIVELY WORK TO REMOVE STRESSORS.

We are going to dig more deeply into the stress epidemic our country is now facing in Chapter Nine. Stress is simply bad news—it can stop or slow down the movement of food through the digestive tract and inhibit the secretion of mucus that is needed to protect the digestive lining. Stress can also lead to digestive problems such as IBS and ulcers.

Research published in the *Journal of Neurogastroenterology and Motility* suggests that stress and depression are related to functional dyspepsia (where the digestive system's peristalsis movement no longer works properly and causes discomfort) and reflux esophagitis (inflammation that damages the esophagus, typically caused by GERD).[303]

For more on stress, see Chapter Nine.

7. QUIT SMOKING AND DRINK LESS ALCOHOL.

Smoking is a terrible idea for many reasons. We all know it leads to lung cancer and other cancers (and Big Tobacco knows it, too, and freely admits it).

But did you know that smoking also hurts your gut?

Smoking weakens the valve at the end of the esophagus, which can lead to acid reflux and heartburn. It also increases the risk of gastrointestinal cancer.[304]

Alcohol doesn't do your gut any favors either. It can interfere with acid secretion, stomach muscles, and nutrient absorption. Its consumption can lead to heartburn, liver problems, and diarrhea. Alcohol also disrupts organ function and digestion. Research published in the *International Journal of Cancer* suggests that cancers of the esophagus, rectum, and liver are strongly related to alcohol consumption.[305]

Now, I do drink wine from time to time, but I don't drink every day, and I make darn sure that my wine is organic and clean crafted with no added sugars. Quality matters!

#GutGoals

The goal when it comes to your digestive tract rests in one word: **resilience.**

Do you want to live your life free from worrying about how you are going to feel after every meal?

There is almost nothing more miserable than having to nit-pick and fret over every single thing you eat. It's no fun to be the friend who has to call ahead to a restaurant to make sure they don't use any gluten or peanuts or dairy or some other random allergy ingredient at the restaurant.

You don't want to have to be the one calling the waiter aside to make sure butter never gets within six feet of your plate, or that their oil is made with *this* and not *that*. All the while, your friends are over there rolling their eyes and thinking to themselves, "Oh, man, why did we invite this party pooper?"

The goal is to be able to eat well but also enjoy life! After all, it's the only one you've got.

The goal with all of this is to live and love and eat good food without having to "pay for it" a few minutes, hours, or even weeks afterward in the form of fatigue, nausea, vomiting, diarrhea, pain, or migraine headaches (and all of the other things that come with food sensitivities and intolerances).

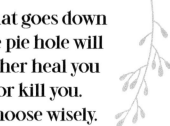

What goes down the pie hole will either heal you or kill you. Choose wisely.

I tell patients every day, you turned these issues on through decades of dysfunction. Most of the time, it's going to take longer than a few weeks (it may take a few months or longer) to reach optimal balance. But I guarantee you what you have "turned on" in your body, you can help turn off if you are diligent enough.

Are there still going to be autoimmune diseases? Yes. Ulcerative colitis? Yes. They say there's no cure for such conditions, but I'm a big believer in fighting for remission. It's a lot of work, and it takes eating lots of the foods that God designed us to eat.

One ingredient, simple foods are the key.

No supplement on earth will make up for a bad diet. You can't take enough pills to fix your heartburn, stomachache, bloating, gas, diarrhea, and constipation. A Pepto-Bismol deficiency is *not* the cause of your diarrhea. A Nexium deficiency is *not* the cause of your heartburn. I should know because I tried every Band-Aid solution under the sun and only made things worse for myself.

Treat the gut with a proactive approach, eat healing foods, avoid inflammatory foods, and you'll enjoy a longer, healthier life. That's why I always say:

What goes down the pie hole will either heal you or kill you. Choose wisely.

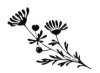

wild & well Rx

Dani Williamson, MSN, FNP

R_x Patient Name: ....

Age: ....   Date: ....

1. Heal your gut, and you heal the majority of many health issues. Reread this chapter if needed.

2. Get something to prop your feet on when you go to the bathroom.

3. Turn around and look at your poop. If it is not a number 4 on the Bristol Stool Chart, start making changes to get it there.

4. Get a good probiotic and take it daily to begin to put good bacteria back into your gut.

5. Pay attention to how you feel after you eat. If you have diarrhea, bloating, gas, gurgling, or constipation, you have a gut issue that most likely stems from diet.

6. Stop smoking asap ("Quit Now" is a great app). Smoking contributes to a leaky gut.

7. Exercise to improve your gut health. Find something you love to do and do it often and with a buddy.

8. Cut down or stop drinking to begin to build the gut lining back. Alcohol does NOT help the gut.

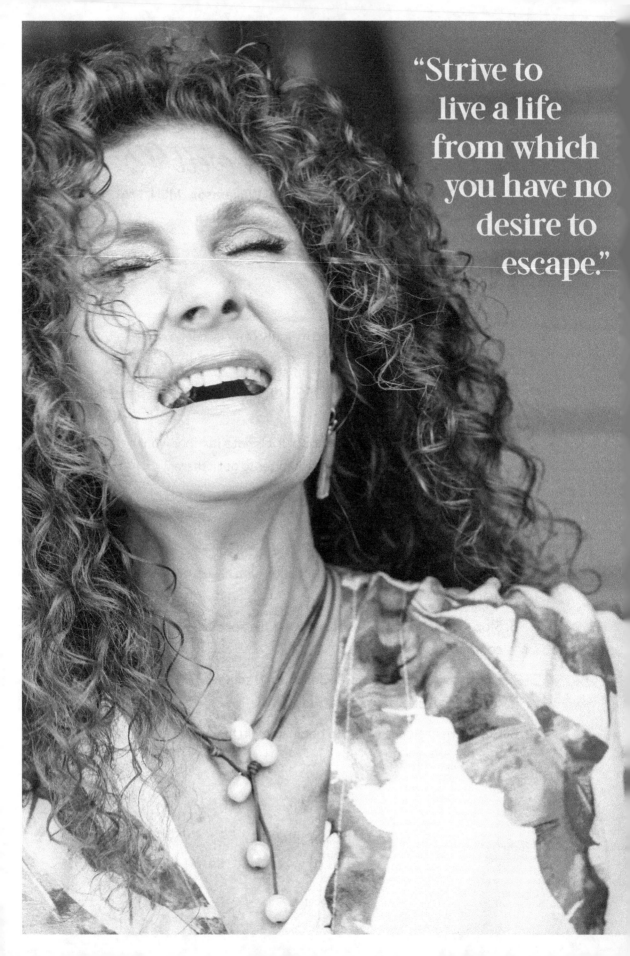

"Strive to live a life from which you have no desire to escape."

de-stress well

"For fast-acting relief, try slowing down."
LILY TOMLIN

Is stress killing you?

We know we're all going to die one day, but did you know that your stress load is one of the largest determinants of how many years you live as well as the *quality* of those years? According to the American Institute of Stress, we're in a real mess. Here are a few indications of just how much of a mess it really is:[306,307]

* Close to 80 percent of people experience stress that affects their physical health.

* Well over 70 percent of people say that stress impacts their mental health.

* Stress does not discriminate by age—high school students cite stress as their number one concern!

* American employers spend over $300 billion every year on healthcare and lost workdays related directly to stress.

* As much as 80 percent of workplace accidents come from stress or stress-related problems, such as being too distracted or excessively tired.

It is estimated that 75 percent of all healthcare provider visits are related to stress.[308] To make matters worse, the leading six causes of death—heart disease, cancer, lung disease, accidents, liver cirrhosis, and suicide—are all linked to stress in some way, thanks in large part to the inflammation caused by a stress response in the body.[309]

Another study showed that 94 percent of American workers report experiencing stress at their workplace in 2019.[310] Can you even imagine what that number is now in a world that has experienced a global pandemic? I bet those numbers are off the charts.

In 2015, researchers at UCLA discovered that in addition to stress, social isolation also triggers cellular changes that result in chronic inflammation, predisposing the lonely to serious physical conditions such as heart disease, stroke, metastatic cancer, and cognitive issues such as Alzheimer's and dementia.[311]

One recent analysis, which pooled data from seventy studies following 3.4 million people over seven years, found that lonely individuals had a 26 percent higher risk of dying.[312]

This figure rose to 32 percent if they lived alone.

If you want to understand the depths of stress and loneliness that we face as a nation, look no further than the benzo and opioid addiction numbers. Quite frankly, they are staggering.

Opioids are responsible for over a hundred deaths every single day.

According to the U.S. Department of Health and Human Services, there are over 14,000 substance abuse facilities in the U.S. alone.[313] This is to help combat the sad reality that more than 760,000 people died from a drug overdose between 1999 and 2018.[314] In 2017, there were 76,994 drug-related deaths, and the CDC estimates that more than 60,000 of these deaths were caused by opioids.[315] Two out of three drug overdose deaths in 2018 involved an opioid.[316]

This will probably come as no surprise, but closely tied to those addiction numbers is the suicide number. The more addictive drugs prescribed, the higher the suicide rate climbs.

If you are feeling stressed or anxious, let me say first that you are *not* alone. In fact, you are so far from alone that it would be a shock to virtually every person you meet if you told them you are *not* stressed.

Stress and anxiety are the norm, not the exception—but that also does not make it okay or healthy to keep living like this.

A Nation of Empty Vessels

When you are stressed and overextended, it's not just you who suffers. You also affect everyone else within your sphere of influence, and that includes not just your family and close friends but also everyone with whom you come into contact!

Inspirational author and speaker Eleanor Brownn said it so well: "Rest and self-care are so important. When you take time to replenish your spirit, it allows you to serve others from the overflow. You cannot serve from an empty vessel."

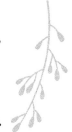

Are you an "empty vessel" right now? If you are, it's time to fill up.

Are you an "empty vessel" right now?

If you are a mom with young kids, or teenage kids, or grandkids…

Or you are raising your grandchildren…

Or you are single but don't want to be…

Or you have a demanding job…

Or you are experiencing a job loss…

Or you've had a recent death in the family…

Or you have ailing parents…

Or you are dealing with personal health issues…

Or you are suffering from an accident…

Or you feel trapped in a tough marriage…

Or you are going through a divorce…

Or you are feeling the aftereffects of a traumatic childhood…

You get the idea.

There are plenty of reasons why you may be running on empty.

You can't serve from an empty vessel, and if you're a woman who is in charge of keeping the household running, let me tell you from experience that all of those people who look to you to keep things operating—they need you to be *healthy* more than they need a ride to soccer practice.

But there are no vacations from being a mother, and we all know this. So, we try and try to keep pouring into our families from that empty vessel.

I have lived it myself, and now I witness it every day in my practice. My patients (these young and not-so-young wives and mothers) are exhausted. They are simply worn out. They have nothing else to give, but they have to keep going.

They don't have a choice, right?

Until one day, the breaking point comes.

There will come a time when you have given all you can give and something else has to give that shouldn't have to. Many times, it's a marriage, or a relationship, or your health.

That is why I say that it's not selfish to put your health first—because you are hands-down a better spouse, partner, parent, son or daughter, employee, or employer when you do.

Detach the Soul Suckers

The first step to prioritize your health is to follow the Wild & Well way discussed in this book. You've got to take in more one-ingredient foods, poop every day, drink lots of clean water, intentionally move each day, get enough sleep every night that you wake up refreshed (remember our first and second sleeps from the sleep chapter), and cultivate friendships.

I know—sounds exhausting!

Well, I have one "hack" for you that makes it all just a little bit less exhausting:

Get rid of the dead weight, otherwise known as the *soul suckers*, in your life today!

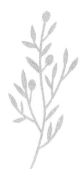

Get rid of the dead weight, otherwise known as the *soul suckers*, in your life today!

You know those people who make you feel worse after you talk to them? Those who have a judgmental word for everything you do? We all have people like this in our lives. But why? What purpose do they serve other than to drag you down into their misery?

There is nothing wrong with getting rid of people. I cut ties with two "friends" about five years ago, and it was one of the best actions I've ever taken to improve my life. The weight I carried was almost instantly lighter. They were women who had been in my life for a long time. I gave and gave, but they were just soul suckers—plain and simple.

I couldn't even tell you how to get in touch with these two ladies today. I deleted them from my phone and blocked them on social media, and I've never looked back.

If someone's presence in your life is not serving you or others, they need to go. It's that simple (but I do know it's not always that easy).

Two of my patients, a hairdresser and a nail tech, actually used the shutdown to purge their client list of toxic soul suckers. They used to complain about certain customers who were never happy. These clients griped, moaned, and carried on about the most trivial things every single time they had their services done.

Well, it just so happened that everyone in the country had to clear their books, and so when things opened back up again, I helped my patients see that they could use that as the perfect opportunity to wipe the slate clean.

I reminded them, "This is your business. You get to choose who you serve."

You don't owe your time to anyone. It's yours—it's within your control. And you need to be more selfish and protective of it.

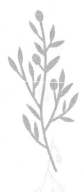

> **You don't owe your time to anyone. It's yours—it's within your control. And you need to be more selfish and protective of it.**

You're worthy of feeling happy, which also means that you're worthy to have people in your life that make you happy and that you enjoy.

Jesus himself set boundaries. He put a little water in between him and the crowds when he needed to. He separated himself from his disciples to go talk to his Father when he needed to.

There's a way to set your business that fits your lifestyle and set boundaries that you're comfortable with and also prevent the wrong people from poisoning the proverbial well within your community.

This process also involves setting expectations for those within your community and with whom you interact. If you don't want to respond to clients or customers on social media, set that expectation. You get to choose!

Just because someone has a social media profile doesn't mean you should communicate with them at all hours of the day. I have never once messaged a doctor, for example, on Facebook or Instagram with a question. If I have a question, I go through the patient portal.

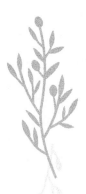

> **There is no rule that says you have to be friends with everybody or that you have to keep the same people in your life forever.**

People have such fluid boundaries now, thanks to social media and our phones and text messaging. I guess they're not even true boundaries anymore if they're fluid, right?

There is no rule that says you have to be friends with everybody or that you have to keep the same people in your life forever.

People change, and that includes you, too! Be willing to keep setting and adjusting those boundaries so that your community remains a place of peace and support rather than drama and toxicity.

There is *nothing* wrong with setting boundaries and cutting out people that are dragging you down into their misery. And that is the key: They want you to be miserable with them. They are unhappy, and they wish you were, too.

At the same time, you also don't want to surround yourself with nothing but "yes men." That's just as unhealthy. You don't need people who will bring you down, but you also don't need people who let you get away with every little thing—every bad attitude, every excuse. You need people on your team who are going to hold you accountable.

> **I'm a big believer in teaching people how to treat you.**

Know your worth, and the first step in figuring that out is to do a *people cleanse*. If someone is causing you stress, then it's okay to remove them or at least limit their influence in your life and stop getting walked on by people. You accomplish this by setting boundaries.

The Best Yes by Lysa Terkeurst is one of the best books I've ever read on setting boundaries. I read the book as a part of a Bible study, and I loved that it wasn't about saying "no" to everything and everyone, but rather it was about what is the best "yes" for you.

Yes, this is a good decision for my family.

Yes, I have the bandwidth for that right now.

Yes, this will bring peace rather than stress into my life.

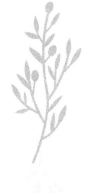

> **I don't know who needs to hear this, but you can still be a phenomenal mother even if you aren't the room mom.**

You must learn what's not good for you and just say yes to the things that are best for you.

I'm a believer in teaching people how to treat you.

Somewhere along the road, we start to believe that part of life is just taking abuse from others. Well, here is a newsflash: That is a lie!

You don't have to feel guilty for saying no. Start getting used to replying with kind but clear honesty, as in, "I can't chair the fall festival this year. I've got a full-time job and a special needs child, but thanks for thinking of me."

I don't know who needs to hear this, but you can still be a phenomenal mother even if you aren't the room mom.

If you are feeling overwhelmed, stop and assess. If your health is declining, take everything off your plate that doesn't involve your personal relationship with the Lord and your partner and/or kids. Slow down on work goals—don't abandon them but get better first. They'll still be there.

> **Strive to live a life from which you have no desire to escape.**

All that "self-care" stuff we hear about is great, and I say a resounding *yes!* to practicing self-care. But don't fall into the trap of making self-care this thing you "escape" to do every once in a while. *Live self-care*, and you don't have to escape from it. You've got a life that you already love.

Strive to live a life from which you have no desire to escape.

"Priority" Isn't Made to be Plural

The idea of achieving a "work-life balance" is so misleading. We all know it's really not possible in our modern world, because let's face it: Work is a part of life. And now, thanks to the large number of people who work from home, the two worlds are inextricably linked—and you do not need to feel guilty about that. Yet, the stress of balancing work and home life are causing such problems. Here are just a few symptoms of our failure to find that elusive and likely mythical balance, according to the American Institute of Stress:[317]

- Businesses lose up to $300 billion yearly as a result of workplace stress.

- Stress causes around one million workers a day to miss work.

- Only 43 percent of U.S. employees think their employers care about their work-life balance.

So, if you can't rely on your business or your boss to prioritize that balance for you (and really, it's not their responsibility anyway), what can you do?

One of the simplest hacks to simply to have an *outlet*—some person or group of people who fully support your need to get things off your chest without making you feel guilty. Maybe that person is your spouse, or maybe it a best friend, sibling, or parent.

Another simple but easy fix is to put the dang phone down. There, I said it because it needed to be said. When you "clock out" at night, take some time away from technology as well.

You can't check your email if you aren't holding your phone.

You can't check your email if you aren't holding your phone.

You are going to have to do something different from what you are doing right now because, if you are like so many others, the stress of life and the lack of perceived balance can lead to depression—and depression is no laughing matter. It causes pure devastation, plain and simple. Here are a few depression and stress stats that will blow your mind:[318]

- Work-related stress and stress-induced depression causes 120,000 deaths every year.

- Stress results in $190 billion in annual healthcare costs.

- Depression leads to $51 billion in annual costs due to absenteeism and $26 billion in yearly treatment costs.

On top of this, did you know that women as a whole feel more committed to their jobs? In fact, this commitment is allegedly one reason why women don't move up the ladder as quickly as men do—they feel a sense of commitment to their position and, therefore, are less prone to vie for new positions. (And don't send me nasty emails about this. You know it's true. So, fight for your rights and ask for that raise, promotion, or corner office)

Speaking of women, we are also shown to be more prone to multitasking because we're better at it (supposedly). However, in the book *Essentialism*, author Greg McKeown talks about the myth of multitasking. Yes, it's a myth!

Although there are always exceptions, it is really impossible for most of us to take on multiple things at once and keep the quality of our activities high.

One fascinating thing I learned a few years ago was that when the word *priority* came into the English language in the 1400s, there was not a plural form of the term. The reason is because *priority* actually means "first."

And how can you have more than one first thing?

It wasn't until the 1900s during the industrial revolution that we pluralized the word priority—and now we have multiple "first things" to do.

We are not supposed to have multiple priorities. Fewer priorities lead to better work, better life, and better connections. So, the whole concept of multitasking—all of it is completely a myth.

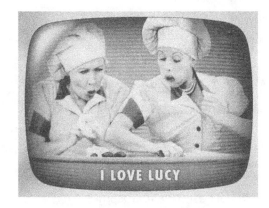

I may be showing my age here, but I have always adored the show "I Love Lucy" starring the legendary Lucille Ball. In one of the most famous episodes, Lucy and her best friend Ethel get a job in a chocolate factory. Ethel and Lucy have one job—to put the chocolates into their wrappers as they pass by on the conveyor belt. At first, the chocolates move slowly along, and they think they've got it covered. But soon, the belt starts to speed up, and before long, they are forced to stuff those chocolates in their shirts, hats, mouths—anywhere to hide the fact that they just can't keep up. It is both hilarious and applicable.

I think we can all relate to this feeling. Life comes at us so quickly, and so we stuff as much down as we can to make room for even more. But, eventually, it all has to spill out somewhere. So, here is how I do priority setting these days.

1. First in my life is God.

2. My family comes next.

3. In all other things, I strive for quality over quantity.

It's ridiculous that the modern world had to add an "s" on to a word just to keep up with the harsh pace of life, and it makes me angry (also sad) when I think about how many different things people think they're required to have to do every day. In reality, loving Jesus, loving your family, and striving to do quality work is really all there is to the vast majority of life.

The Three Magic Words

At some point during the day, you'll need to eat some food that'll make your body feel good. How complex those meals are? That's entirely up to you. At some point, you also need to move your body and drink water. Shower if and when you must and take good care of your teeth (since it's a one-of-a-kind, irreplaceable collection)!

Then, if you can fit in anything else, it's all bonus.

Automate, Eliminate, Delegate.

My mom's dementia? It's a part of my daily life, but it's not something I can control. Therefore, I have to learn how to live and deal with it. It's not going anywhere, and there is no head-in-the-sand approach that works for dealing with cognitive decline.

But I'll tell you what: There is a whole lot of stuff I CAN control. One of the easiest shortcuts to achieving control is called "AED," which stands for:

Automate, Eliminate, Delegate.

These three words are such keys to keeping my life operating on *my* terms. Just like the AED device at the gym or the mall, this AED can also bring you back to life!

For the most part, we're in control of our stress and how we manage our stress. What is it that's keeping us continually stressed out? Where's the barrier for us, for not taking control of our life and setting boundaries and eliminating, automating, delegating?

My friend, prolific author, and leadership development authority Michael Hyatt is the one who first introduced me to the AED concept. Here is a brief summary:

First, *automate* as much as possible in your life. From grocery shopping to banking and bill pay and so much more. Everything you can automate… take it off your plate! Stop writing checks. Stop going to grocery store and order online. My daughter Ella works at Whole Foods and shops for people, and it's got to be one of the best tools ever for busy working families!

Now, going to the grocery store is relaxing for me and also a chance to network and connect (I always see patients there), but if grocery shopping is stressful for you, automate with a shopping app such as Instacart, Shipt, or Prime Now.

If I was raising little kids in today's world, I would automate my shopping. You wouldn't catch me in the grocery store for any amount of money. There was nothing worse for me than going to shop for groceries when my kids were young, and their moods were unpredictable (and I was exhausted). I left the store with the cart full and two screaming kids in my arms more than once.

Next, *delegate* things that can be delegated. Lift your finger off just enough so that you can start to let go and let others help. Trying to do it all yourself—it's just not working, is it?

Finally, and admittedly this one can be the toughest one for many—*eliminate*. Eliminate the stuff that doesn't matter. Take a look at everything with honest intention and get rid of what really doesn't matter and doesn't bring you joy.

I believe that for the most part, we create our own stress. Yes, life brings us stress in the form of things we can't control (such as a worldwide pandemic), but we create a lot of stress ourselves. We don't loosen the reins and we are hard on our spouses because they don't dress the kids the way we would ("Can't he see those shoes don't match?") or feed the kids the way we would ("You mean you let them have a fruit rollup right before lunch?").

At some point, you're going to have to loosen the reins a bit—and when you do finally give over some of the control, guess what? The kids are going to be alright. Someone else may not do it the way you would, but if it gets done, then it's still a win! I wish I had seen this clearly when I was raising my children.

We have to do things that are sustainable.

We have to find balance.

Now, if you are an all or nothing person like me, that's a tough ask. The word *moderation* is not a useful word to me. I'm usually an all or nothing kind of gal, but I'm working on it. I have yet to find that balance on a consistent basis, but I continue to strive for it every single day. I am in my mid-fifties and trust me—I am still becoming a master at "AED'ing" my life. I only wish I had started thirty years ago. But, hey, better late than never, right?

If and when you do commit to letting others help, you are also going to have to make another pledge at the same time—to stop nagging. Nagging may feel necessary ("How else are they going to know?") but, really, it's not.

For the most part, women are the naggers. Yes, there are a few men who nag, but it's primarily a role filled by women. That's hard medicine right there, but it needed to be said.

Ladies, just remember that good men—men that are worth keeping—are simple. Dr. Laura Schlesinger has always said it best: They want good food, good sex, and to protect you. It's as simple as that. If you will give them those three things, they are putty in your hands for the rest of your life. If I ever get married again, I will be handing out, *The Proper Care and Feeding of Husbands*, to every person at my wedding. That book made me think, "Wow, spot on, Dr. Laura," over and over again. It's a game changer. Order it, and let me know what you think.

Notice what did not make the list? Constant nagging. There is almost nothing more emasculating to a man than for his woman to be badgering him about this or that, day-in and day-out.

If you're a homemaker, and your partner comes home after a tough day at work, as much stress as you faced that day, your partner faced his fair share, too. His stress looked different from yours, but also think about the fact he had to face the cold, cruel world while you did your work from the comfort of home.

Give that man a little breathing room when he comes home, and everyone will be better for it. Men don't want their tail chewed out the second they open the front door.

Marriages can be destroyed through nagging. I've seen it happen. Don't let a good marriage fizzle out because of nagging.

The Straightforward Solution

In Chapter Six, we discussed the fact that the body can't tell the difference between good stress and bad stress. It could be a death in the family or wedding planning.

Stress is stress to the body.

Stress is stress to the body.

Let's review the basic types of stress we experience:

- **Eustress**—"good" stress from activities and events such as marriage, new baby, new friends, job promotion, graduation, and even winning the lottery.

- **Distress**—"bad" stress from activities and events such as accidents, sickness, relationship problems, financial stress, and negative feelings.

- **Acute Stress**—stress the body feels in any fight or flight situation. The body prepares to defend itself, and it takes about ninety minutes for the metabolism to return to normal afterwards.

- **Chronic Stress**—ongoing stress that comes with daily living and includes bills, kids, jobs. This is the stress we tend to ignore or push down. Left uncontrolled, this stress adversely affects your health in many ways.

No matter what kind of reality you are experiencing—good or bad—your brain believes whatever you say. That means when you are going through a stressful situation, *you* decide how your body interprets it. The next time you are faced with adversity or a challenge, try speaking words of life into existence, as in, "I know this looks bad, but it's okay. This is something that will make us better."

Encourage your body! There is a lot of science to support affirmations.

- Science has shown that people suffering from anxiety and depression find affirmations reminding them that they aren't "crazy" and that their depression is not permanent helps them recover more quickly.[319]

- Positive affirmations also appear to reduce resistance to change, especially as it relates to health behavior changes.[320]

The bottom line is we live in a stressed-out world, and, within that world, we live in the most stressed out country on earth. Over half of the American population experiences stress during the day, and that is a staggering 20 percent higher than the world average of 35 percent.[321]

What I also have discovered as a startlingly common theme is that, for the most part, people hate their jobs. If this is the case, then what in the world keeps them from changing their reality?

The obvious answer is fear of change.

The word *change*—people really tend to hate that word in general. It represents work and effort and pain and also the unknown.

Let's say you are stuck in a job you hate, and someone says, "Then go back to school and learn how to do something else."

People who are averse to change will be quick with the responses (excuses) that sound like:

1. That is too expensive.

2. I'm too old now.

3. I don't have any extra time.

> **Don't tell me it's impossible to change your career, because I've done it multiple times and never looked back.**

I get it—change often requires complicated solutions. But since when is "complicated" and "impossible" the same thing?

Don't tell me it's impossible to change your career, because I've done it multiple times and never looked back.

Even after I became an FNP and started loving what I do, I was working at a practice that became highly stressful. One day, the office manager called me in and said, "You know you're going to have to leave, right? Because this job is killing you."

Guess what? She was right, and I did! And because of that choice, I ended up starting my own business, and now I have my dream job and the best boss in the world (me). I will say that my former boss was pretty incredible himself. He is the reason I do what I do, and he taught me functional medicine from the ground up—and for that I am eternally grateful to Dr. Dan Kalb.

Don't tell me you can't do it. Yes, you can.

I was in an unhealthy marriage. I did what I had to do to get out and make a happier life for my kids and me. I did what I had to do to pull myself up from the bootstraps.

Fear doesn't have to stop you.

I've been scared so many times throughout my life. But I've never been too scared to make the change. I just can't imagine fear paralyzing me enough to leave me feeling stuck and miserable.

Whether it's work, an abusive marriage, or a toxic relationship, there is always a way out and through. There is not even a set rule that says you have to maintain a relationship with a toxic family member no matter what. If your uncle or mother-in-law or brother is creating stress in your life, limit their influence. You get to make those decisions for yourself, not them or your spouse or society.

Some people really are programmed to be paralyzed by fear, to assume that things won't work out and, therefore, what's the point in even trying? That is not how I'm wired, as I seem to have an innate *growth* mindset. Sadly, there also seems to be plenty of people who have an innate *fixed* mindset—and that is why there is so much work and relationship dissatisfaction. People who have an innate fixed mindset tend to marry the first decent person who comes along or take the "easy" job instead of waiting for what they really want.

We're talking about the "low hanging fruit" people.

If that describes you, don't choose to be insulted by these words. Instead, choose to be motivated by them and by the knowledge that there is *always* a way. ALWAYS.

There is a way to retrain your brain. "Neuroplasticity" is the ability of neural networks in the brain to change through growth and reorganization. In layman's terms, here is what it boils down to:

You can, in fact, teach an old dog new tricks.

The last thing I want to do is make you feel stressed about feeling stressed or feel guilty because there are people or things you can't cut from your life right now. That seems a bit counterproductive, so I'll just say this…

You can, in fact, teach an old dog new tricks.

Tomorrow is a new day, and when the sun rises, you get a fresh chance to do things a little differently. When you wake up in the morning, there are three places you can choose to live: the past, the future, or the present.

You have people who live in *regret*, and that's living in the **past**. You have people who live in *fear*, and that's living in the **future**. Then you have those very few people who live *consciously* with a growth mindset, and they live in the **present**.

If we could all live like that third one, we'd be a lot happier.

It's like exercise. It's like eating well. Yeah, it's gonna take some work. That's life—so get used to it. If you don't like it, that's okay, too.

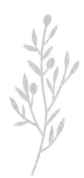

At some point, you either refuse to change or you change. You just have those two options.

At some point, you either refuse to change or you change. You just have those two options.

Maybe you go to bed each night with grand plans for the next day. You are going to start eating well, work out, tell loved ones how you really feel, spend more time with the kids, and so much more. Well, what if tomorrow is the day when you finally start taking action? Just think of the possibilities!

The 2020 pandemic reinforced a lot of people's tendency to live in the future. What if I get sick? What if I come in contact with someone who is sick? What if I infect someone? What if I can't find any toilet paper? What if my kid can't ever attend school in person again? What if I lose my job? What if I can't find another one?

I have a newsflash for you. You are, in fact, going to die one day. The chances of it being from COVID-19 are slim. In fact, the chances are much higher that heart disease or cancer will be your cause of death, and the way most people stress-ate during the lockdown only increased the odds of dying from a lifestyle-related disease. I was so hoping people would use the time during the 2020 lockdown and after to start learning how to cook, find new recipes to make, get the kids in the kitchen, and exercise more. Sadly, so many of my patients and friends tell me they opted for eating comfort food, moving less (not more), and being way too stressed to spend time teaching their kids how to cook.

Should the fact that you are mortal and will one day breathe your last breath change the way you live life? It really shouldn't.

And, yet, we default to the worst every single time. This *worst-case-scenario* mentality is wreaking havoc on our mental and physical health. From over-eating and anxiety to depression and suicide, the "what ifs" are killing us.

When I'm really overwhelmed, I do a few simple things that, when combined, can go a long way toward taking my focus from of the past or future and back into the present:

- Take deep breaths.

- Turn off my phone.

- Pray.

- Laugh with a friend.

- Slow down and do something enjoyable.

Of course, the worldwide pandemic taught us the slowing down our schedules and *actually* relaxing are two different things. Some of my patients spent more time with their kids during lockdown than they had in years. Is this a good thing or a bad thing? I'm hoping it was good and that you love being around your family. If you don't, could it be that you are all too busy doing life to really know and appreciate each other?

Stress is hard to control. In fact, trying to control it can be stressful. I pray that you will find ways to live in the present and enjoy each moment just a little more.

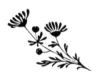

wild & well Rx

Dani Williamson, MSN, FNP

R℞   Patient Name: ....

Age: ....   Date: ....

1. Live in the present. Don't live in the past or the future. Your life will be much fuller and happier when you choose to live in the here and now.

2. Get rid of the soul suckers in your life!! Just do it and thank me later.

3. Read *The Best Yes* by Lysa Terkerst. It was a game changer for me.

4. Create a life for yourself from which you don't feel the need to escape, and make a life that incorporates self-care into it.

5. AED your life! It just may save it. Automate, eliminate, and delegate everything you can.

6. Read *The Proper Care and Feeding of Husbands* whether you are married or not. It's hard medicine, but, wow, it's a life-changing book.

7. Take inventory of what you want to change and then change it. You are not stuck.

8. Put your stressors into perspective. If you died today, would those stressors from yesterday even matter?

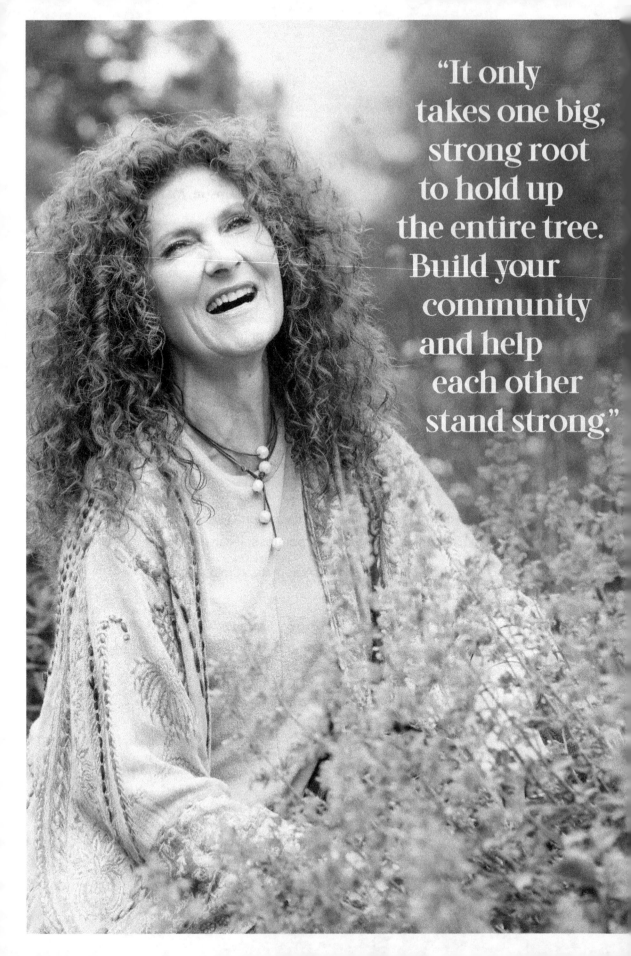

"It only takes one big, strong root to hold up the entire tree. Build your community and help each other stand strong."

commune well

*"Friends are people who know you really well
and like you anyway."*

GREG TAMBLYN

My job as a practitioner of functional medicine is *not* to consider the symptoms and treat accordingly. That's surface stuff. That's lazy. That's also a big part of what's gotten us into the mess we're in now with our health as a nation.

My job is to find out what's *really* going on with my patients—to dig down and find the root of their issue or, let's be honest, issues... with an *s*. Then, we do the lab work to further substantiate what we've uncovered and fill in the gaps to come up with a treatment plan.

Those are the basics of functional medicine, and it's a far superior form of medicine over modern (allopathic) medicine in many ways.

Now, you and I may never meet face to face, but I want you to know that I wrote this book to bridge the gap for you, and to encourage you to keep digging until you find the root of your issues. However, I also need to say this:

I am *not* here to hold your hand. It's not my job to walk this entire journey with you, telling you each step to take.

As a functional medicine practitioner, I believe that the mental and emotional aspects of health are as important as physical health. However, because I'm not a trained psychologist, a pastor, or a close friend or family member, I'm not the right person to help you through each psychological hurdle.

As nice as it would be to have someone tell you every move to make and when, that's just not how it works. No one provider or even friend or loved one can or should be that person for you.

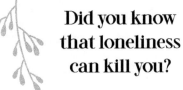

Did you know that loneliness can kill you?

God is your biggest advocate, first and foremost. Then, you are *supposed* to be able to rely on family. Sadly, many people do not have that luxury.

That is where community comes in!

If you think this is all just the icing on the cake of this book, you'd be wrong. You can eat well, sleep well, move well, poop well, and de-stress well, but if you don't laugh and live your life surrounded by others and exist as a lone wolf with no support, how is that *living well*?

Did you know that sadness can make you sick?

Did you know that loneliness can kill you?

Sadness, loneliness, and isolation are silent killers, but are you ever going to see those listed as a cause of death on any death certificate? Of course not, but we know darn good and well that they affect every aspect of our health.

We saw it all too plainly during the 2020 pandemic and subsequent lockdowns and separation that followed. We read the reports of teens taking their lives due to loneliness and isolation. We heard about elderly patients (or maybe even had our own family members) in nursing homes who would rather die than go one more day without getting a hug from their family.

I speak from experience on this. My mother is in an assisted living facility thanks to the ravages of Alzheimer's. The original lockdown in the spring of 2020 almost killed her. Her mobility, cognitive function, and even bladder control all rapidly declined. She can no longer walk independently, has to wear "padded panties" as we call them, and her memory worsened significantly. During a second lockdown, she contracted COVID-19, and I had to manage her care from the outside—literally from her apartment window.

Here is an excerpt from an article reporting the devastating effects on so many of the elderly members of our society:[322]

> Seclusion and depression, whether caused by fear of contracting the virus or facility restrictions, has become such a problem among the elderly, death certificates now read cause of death as "isolation/failure to thrive related to COVID-19 restrictions."

Our feelings, our emotions, and how they physically affect every organ and system in the body is as real as the nose on my face, and that is why community simply *must* be a part of any respectable functional medicine regimen.

Building a community of true friends that give you the support you need will never happen by accident, and it will never happen without a ton of work and face time.

But wow, it's so worth it!

Now, as of the writing of this book, I'm single. I'd love for that to change one day, but I have to say that, in many ways, being single is what made me realize the importance of building a thriving community. I don't know what I'd do without my neighbors, my friends, and my online connections, and

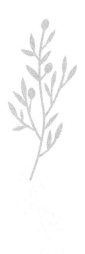

When you take the time to connect with others, you create sounding boards and you find the resources you need to heal—emotionally, physically, sexually, mentally, and spiritually.

that is why I try harder than anyone I know to actively cultivate those groups and give others what they need with the hope that they will return the favor or, even better, "pay it forward" by supporting someone else.

When you take the time to connect with others, you create sounding boards and you find the resources you need to heal—emotionally, physically, sexually, mentally, and spiritually.

Functional medicine practitioners can help you uncover or bring to light what underlying issues may be contributing to the state of your health. It is then up to you to build the kind of community that provides you with the EXACT kind of support you need to thrive again!

Jesus Modeled Community

Throughout my life, I've always unintentionally created a community that I wasn't even aware of until I stepped back one day in awe of what I had. Thanks to a highly stressful childhood and a family that was just not very close, I tended to gravitate toward others who were kind and good and gave me many of the things I did not have growing up.

My "core" set of friendships—my inner circle—have been there for decades. There are five of us, and we might as well be blood related because we are closer than the closest sisters.

One of the best examples of community is Jesus' disciples. It's your crew—your squad, your tribe—that will always be there for you. Within Jesus' twelve, he too had an inner circle (the three who seemed to have enjoyed the closest relationship with him): Peter, John, and John's brother James. They were the ones who had the most conversations with him and were selected by Jesus to accompany him on special occasions.

John enjoyed an even more special affinity than the others as was even referred to as "the disciple whom Jesus used to love." Peter was certainly right up there as well. In Matthew 16:18, Jesus told Peter, "And I say also unto thee, that thou art Peter, and upon this rock I will build my church; and the gates of hell shall not prevail against it."

Throughout his time in his ministry, Jesus appreciated and demonstrated the fact that community is so important! And we're not talking about your "yes men." That's not what community is.

Your community is made up of people who hold you to the truth. They also tell you the truth, whether you want to hear it or not. They speak truth into you, and they're the ones standing there when all heck breaks loose around you.

Your real community, and particularly your core group, is there with you even if you make a few (or a lot of) mistakes. When I had an affair decades ago and my life imploded all around me, everyone in my life scattered like the wind in 42 directions—that is, except for my core people. They were the ones still standing there when the smoke cleared.

I'm extremely blessed to have four women who are there for me through thick and thin. That's true abundance! In fact, you are blessed if you just have *one* person who is your root.

It only takes one big, strong root to hold up the entire tree.

> **It only takes one big, strong root to hold up the entire tree.**

Outside of your core inner circle, you have your larger community, which can look very different for everyone. One of the arms of my community is the Hashimoto's support group I've been running for almost a decade. During 2020, we were no longer able to meet in person, and it wasn't until it was taken away that I realized just how much I'd come to depend on that group of people.

The members felt the same way I did, and they begged me to start the meetings again. For some of them, it was their only community, and, oh, how they needed it.

During Summer 2020, the lockdowns prompted me to do something I should have done years ago. I started a weekly neighborhood cookout, and it quickly became the most important thing I did each week. It was a lot of work, but, boy, it was worth it for each and every one of us.

We'd meet outside, bring lots of food, and fellowship with each other for hours (from a safe distance). All these years of living next to each other, and we'd just passed by and waved. We are a great neighborhood that all knew each other before the lockdown, but we didn't truly *know* each other until week after week, we met and laughed, cried, and learned about each other. We stopped and talked and got to know each other better, and the relationships we made will impact the rest of our lives and have changed us all for the better.

Women Set the Tone

I remember years ago, coming home from nurse practitioner school exhausted, overwhelmed, and defeated every day. I was the oldest student by a long shot for most of the program. I was divorced and on food stamps, scraping together pennies and dimes to survive. One of my kids was struggling in every class and was being bullied. On top of it all, I had to drive the kids up to Kentucky every other weekend so they could see their dad—a man who was still extremely bitter against me at the time.

It was a mess.

As soon as I'd walk in the house, one of the kids would send me into a tailspin. I yelled. I said terrible things. I remember once saying to Ella, "I'm never upset during the day. As soon as I come home, you act ugly, and it sets me off."

If Jesus had ever suddenly appeared before me in those moments, I would have been so humiliated and horrified at the things I said. Of course, he *was* there, even though I couldn't see him. We would all do well to remember that, wouldn't we?

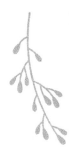

> **That is because women like that have no margin in their life. There's no room for error.**

In truth, my kids weren't acting "ugly" or anything else. All they really wanted was for their mom to pay attention to them.

So many women can relate to this sentiment. They know they shouldn't lose their temper over the slightest thing, but they feel inches away from spiraling at any moment.

That is because women like that have no margin in their life. There's no room for error.

They're on that hamster wheel with no idea how to slow it down.

The problem is that when the momma's unhappy and unhealthy, she is far too irritable and short tempered, and just plain unpleasant to be around.

The bottom line is when you're not happy with your life, the people who pay the most are your family. Every week, I listen to mothers in my office tell me how unhappy they are. They're not happy with their husbands, their jobs, their work in the home, their life situation, their bank account, their weight, their kids' attitudes.

They're barely treading water.

This is a treacherous attitude because as women, we set the tone for our home. The husband may be the head of the household, but as the mother said in the classic movie, *My Big Fat Greek Wedding*, the woman is the neck, and she can turn the head any way she wants. The mom sets the direction.

The health of the household? It's on us. Our attitude becomes the attitude of the entire home.

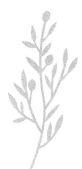

The health of the household? It's on us. Our attitude becomes the attitude of the entire home.

So, if this is all true (and it is), how do we prevent the hamster wheel to keep us on the run? I'm afraid it's an answer that most won't like, because it requires the same thing it takes to eat right and reclaim your health. You have to consciously plan. You have to meet the day head on rather than let the day dictate how it will treat you.

"What is my menu going to look for the day (even better, for the week)?"

"What is the schedule for the day?"

"What is my top priority today?"

"Have I overcommitted? What can I delegate?"

"What can I eliminate altogether?"

"What small thing can I do to make this day special?"

At the end of the day, there are really only two conclusions. Will you fall into bed, feeling like you ran in a hamster wheel? Or will you lie down in your bedroom sanctuary, content in the knowledge that at least a few times during the day, you took the time to stop and smell a few roses?

It's up to you.

It really is all up to you.

Practice an Attitude of Gratitude

Gratitude has become a buzzword in today's motivational coaching scene, but don't let that distract you from an indisputable truth: *Being grateful improves your health!*

Giving grace and being grateful are anti-inflammatory.

Being grateful increases your serotonin and your dopamine, which are your feel-good neurotransmitters.

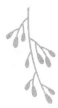

Giving grace and being grateful are anti-inflammatory.

It also decreases anxiety and depression.

It lowers blood pressure, and it improves your energy.

Now, we can certainly all be grateful when things are good. But what about when they aren't?

When you are stuck in your head, feeling sorry for yourself, can't seem to find any answers, or just struggling, go volunteer. Give back to someone who needs help. I always feel better when I step outside of my own head and do something for somebody else.

The research is clear: Giving back changes your attitude. It makes you more grateful. You'll be grateful for your hot shower. Grateful for every bit of food. Grateful to be able to turn on working lights in your home.

I realize that life isn't always fair, and it's also not easy. But being grateful for even the smallest things in life will do wonders for your health, and it can also change your attitude and make you realize that maybe, just maybe, things are not as bad as they seem. Consider this:

* That job you have? I know it may not feel this way, but millions of other people would love to have it.

* That kid who is in a difficult season? Think of the people who can't have kids.

* That spouse you complain about every day? Let me tell you there are millions of people who'd love to have a spouse just like him or her. I know I'd love to have a man and call him all mine!

Be consciously grateful for the little things rather than just the obvious blessings. I speak my gratitude aloud every single day, and I mention everything I can think to include!

> "Good Lord, thank you for my heart and my lungs. Thank you for my brain and my working organs. Thank you for giving me a body that is designed to heal itself. Thank you for my home and my fantastic kids. And thanks for my legs! There are people on this earth whose legs don't work or who don't even have legs at all."

I don't know why, but I'm especially grateful for my legs. They are body parts that I feel like get taken for granted, and so I acknowledge mine as much as possible. The cellulite, the flab, and the jiggly thighs—grateful for all of it.

Once you start to make gratitude a part of your daily life, it will rub off on your kids as well.

My kids grew up going to Goodwill, Walmart, and secondhand clothing stores. I'll never forget the day my daughter Ella told my wealthy (but also kind and gracious) friend Billie, who was wearing a shirt she got from Target, "Oh, my gosh. We don't go to Target. It's too expensive."

Billie and I still laugh about that.

There's nothing wrong with telling your kids, "We don't have the money for that." Even though I wasn't happy about being on foods stamps and a medical card when my kids were growing up, I am grateful that they now have the mindset that Target is expensive. Both of my kids still shop at Goodwill and go first to the sale racks when they shop.

I'm grateful that I've struggled, and saved money, and lived below my means. It makes me so grateful for what I now have. The bonus is when you live below your means, you're able to help more people. When you spend less money than you make, you can give more money away.

Those are the kinds of actions that build a sense of community.

Grateful people are happier, healthier, and more whole. Grateful people eat better, sleep better, move better, and poop better. Their stress level is lower.

I think gratefulness is good for us in *every* possible way, and I encourage you to start practicing it each morning and throughout the day. Be grateful for the big and the small and everything in between.

Community in a Post-Pandemic World

I don't know what community is ultimately going to look like in a post-pandemic world, but I know what I sense about it. I feel strongly that we're not intended to live in seclusion.

God did not design us for isolation. He designed us for interaction and for community. In searching for more on this topic, I stumbled onto an article from Dave Ramsey on community (with permission from his wife to include this excerpt):[323]

God didn't intend for us to live in isolation. He specifically designed us to crave—and thrive in—relationship with others. We're our best selves when we're experiencing life's highs and lows with others. That means everyone, whether you're single or married, needs community.

Don't take it from us though. The Bible has a lot to say about this topic! Here are four reasons the Bible tells us community is so important:

1. **Community is encouraging.** Being in community gives you the chance to be around people at different stages of their faith journey—and to bear their burdens alongside them (Galatians 6:2). That's awesome, because everyone has something to teach and to learn.

2. **Community is fun.** Community should never feel boring or forced. In fact, it should be the exact opposite. Psalm 133:1 (NIV) tells us, "How good and pleasant it is when God's people live together in unity!"

3. **Community attracts the Holy Spirit.** The Bible says the Holy Spirit is present whenever believers gather together (Matthew 18:20). A great example of this was the early church of Acts, which made a habit of meeting together, eating together, and worshiping together. As a result, "the Lord added to their number daily those who were being saved" (Acts 2:46–47 NIV).

4. **Community fosters love.** Paul held love above all else in his letter to the Corinthians. And he did the same with his letter to the Colossians: "Bear with each other and forgive one another if any of you has a

> grievance against someone. Forgive as the Lord forgave you. And over all these virtues put on love, which binds them all together in perfect unity" (Colossians 3:13–14 NIV).
>
> Bonus reason: Community is life-giving and essential to following Christ. Scripture says that's because we're better together than we are alone (Romans 12:4–5).

The message is clear: We have to become more intentional with building our relationships, just like I did when I started the weekly cookout with neighbors.

The lockdown hashtag that started in 2020 (#alonetogether) is contradictory. Those two words are simply not meant to coexist.

Studies show that when people don't have physical touch, it leads to depression and more. At my mom's assisted living home, physical touch is no longer allowed. No hugs. No sitting next to one another at dinner.

How is that okay?

If you are severely immune compromised, then you have to do what's right for you. But for most of us, it is more harmful to stay isolated inside than it is to go out and practice safe health practices while being around others. Wash your hands, cover your mouth when you cough, and don't go out when you are sick. Use common sense.

I am not a leading authority on infectious diseases, but I've seen the survival rates for viral infections, and I've also seen the devastation that isolation brings, and, for me personally, it's worth the risk to take the right safety measures and then go out and be with my community—my support system.

We are just now beginning to see the mental health repercussions of this new era of isolation, and it's overwhelming.

We know that isolated and lonely people have a higher suicide rate, and that has certainly shown itself to be true in 2020. During that year, suicide rates increased (we won't know the true numbers for another few years). Phone calls to crisis hotlines were up over 800 percent compared to recent years.

The suicide rates continue to climb, and tragically, the 10- to 13-year-olds are a group of children that are dying by suicide at alarming rates—more than other age ranges right now. Is it peer pressure on social media? I think that's a large part of it, compounded by the fact that kids can't be average anymore.

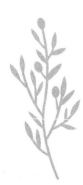

> **People are scared of "average" now because "average" doesn't get you into college or look good on Instagram.**

Average doesn't get you into college. Average doesn't look good on Instagram.

Bullying is also on the rise. One of my kids was bullied and one was not, and I can tell you that bullying destroys lives. If you're not just another part of the herd, you're picked *out* and picked *on* until you either move, crack, or fold.

Community in a post-pandemic world should be even more important to us than ever. Zoom serves its purpose. Facetime is better than nothing. Facebook, Instagram, and the like—they all have value. But nothing replaces person-to-person, face-to-face, eyeball-to-eyeball contact.

My Instagram and Facebook communities are a great supplement, but online groups and virtual friends are not substitutes for the real thing. That's similar to what I tell my patients about supplements, which is that supplements are great additions *to* but not substitutes *for* eating well. Unless you're eyeball-to-eyeball with someone, there's so much that can be misconstrued.

Online community is simply not enough for our species to thrive. We need each other! We need hugs, and we need to show up for others and be there when they are weak. I truly believe that no man or woman is an island nor should they ever be forced to be.

You Deserve to Be Wild & Well

We have spent decades with our priorities flipped upside down. Our jobs, our kids, our partner, our friends, and even our laundry often gets put before what should be first.

And that is God.

When things get put before Christ, we end up with chaos, disconnection, and distance between the people we love. If you're not a Christian, I can't speak to that, because I am. I simply know that whenever God is not first and foremost in my life, that's when the chaos starts.

After God comes your spouse, if you are married. And if you are married or have ever been married, you know that "getting married" is the easy part. The rubber really meets the road when the children are born, the job is lost, the bills pile up, the hormones start to tank, and the libido is gone.

One lesson I preach to every one of my tank-on-empty moms is that children are third, after God and after your spouse. Those kids need to see Mom and Dad side by side, always. You are the center. You are together. You were Husband and Wife—a dynamic duo—before you became Mom and Dad. And if things work out as planned, it'll just be the two of you again after the kids are grown and independent.

But there's the other side, too. I have two divorce attorney patients who say they could *not* stop working during lockdown. After a few months trapped inside together, more and more couples realized they didn't like each other anymore.

How truly tragic and heartbreaking that is to me. However, I feel strongly you can avoid this fate by keeping your relationship with your spouse in second place just behind God. I also had another attorney tell me she had a few clients reconcile during the pandemic.

But please—I'm begging you—before you try to fix any worldly relationship—take the time to fix *you*. Do that and the whole family heals. As the central focus of your home (if you are a woman), you are the barometer that indicates the health of the whole home and everyone in it.

You are worthy to put on your oxygen mask first.

When you do that, you change not only your life but the whole trajectory of your family's life—and even your grandchildren's lives! How incredible is that?

You'll also be able to cultivate a much more dynamic, loving, and enduring community.

If you do all of that, you'll start to fully pursue the life that God designed you to live, which one that is rich in full and abundant health. I don't think it can get any better than that.

People heal when they have community. So, do the work to find other people who think like you. Other people who can help you along your healing journey, whatever that may be. Whether it's your church group, your neighbors, your crew from college, Weight Watchers, Al-Anon, AA, a women's group, or a men's group. You need people to lift you up, give you hard truths that sometimes you don't want to hear, and stand beside you when the smoke clears.

You heal when you have community.

About seven years ago, I started a community on Facebook. It's a private group called *Inside Out—Healing from Within*. At over 10,000 strong as of 2021, we are an unbelievable community of people who are just like you. We are looking to heal ourselves from the inside out. I started this group as a safe place for my patients to ask questions to each other without feeling anxiety. Unbelievably, people from all over the world started asking to join the community.

I recently ran into someone while in the grocery, and she told me, "Inside Out is my go-to for all things health related." It made my heart happy to hear that.

"What do I do to begin healing?"

"How do I start?"

You can ask any question under the sun. It's a safe, private place to share and ask. I have a $29 course on my website, "Inflammation Is the Devil," that is designed for anyone who is not sure where to begin. It covers everything that I discuss with patients during their first in-office visit in an easy-to-digest format. The course also includes my six steps to healing and what causes inflammation, the root of all chronic lifestyle disease **(DaniWilliamson.com/Wild)**.

I also have endless hours of information available through my *Sunday Night Services* (they air live every Sunday night at 6:00 p.m. CST) on everything from detoxing and autoimmune disease to sleeping better and restoring your sex life with your spouse! I am blessed to have many prominent health leaders as guests on my Sunday Night Services to share their knowledge as well. Those Sunday Night Services are on my Dani Williamson Wellness page, and you can watch live or the next day when they are transferred to my YouTube Channel of the same name. I have hundreds of videos for you to watch and learn from.

Then, of course, there is my website, DaniWilliamson.com, which has everything that you need. There are plenty of ways to get in touch with me and to get plugged in to different communities. I also have online courses and plenty of free educational videos.

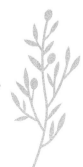

If you sign up for my newsletter at DaniWilliamson.com, you will get weekly updates and health articles.

If you sign up for my newsletter at **DaniWilliamson.com**, you will get weekly updates and health articles.

I also do brief, five-minute-long educational talks on most days on various topics on my *Dani Williamson Wellness* Facebook page.

My Instagram page @daniwilliamsonwellness has a daily recipe, video, or educational graphic on various health-related topics.

If you're new to this healing journey but ready to take that next step—and if you really want to decrease inflammation, eat well, poop well, sleep well, move well, relax well, and connect well—then you have to step out of the boat and walk toward help.

I know how hard it is, and I also know that of all the disciples, Peter was the *only* disciple who took the bold step to get out of that boat. And guess what, his faith paid off in a big way—he walked on water!

You can as well. I believe that with everything in me, and I know how to help you do that. I have all kinds of resources to help you.

I'm honored and thrilled that I get to do what I love every single day. I'm also humbled and amazed by the fact that I feel good. I sleep well. I wake up bright eyed and bushy tailed each morning. My stomach doesn't hurt anymore. I'm not depressed. I don't itch every day. My joints don't hurt any more.

I know that your journey can have a similar story.

I also know that what I'm asking you to do is not easy.

That is why you need to cultivate your community. You also need a trusted provider who can walk along beside you, someone who can help you begin to realize that you don't have an "eating problem." In reality, what you may have is a *thinking problem*. And really, you could interject anything into that conclusion:

> "I don't have a _____ (drug, alcohol, weight, anxiety) problem. I have a thinking problem."

Of course, I am not downplaying *real* conditions with an undeniable physiological component such as chronic disease, depression, anxiety, and addictions. What I am saying is that without acknowledging the spiritual and emotional components to those issues, true healing may never take place.

You need someone (or better yet, a whole group of someones!) to help you rethink how you're doing things. *That* is when you begin to heal, walk the journey that you're designed to walk, and live the life that you were designed to live, which is in true and optimal health.

No one wants to be "normal" anyway.

We all want to be optimal!

We want to live our lives freely—and let's be honest....

We'd all love to get a little Wild & Well.

I hope you enjoyed our journey together. Find me on Facebook, Instagram, or YouTube, or reach out on my website. I look forward to hearing your story and how you reclaimed the health and happiness that God meant for you to experience.

May the Lord bless you and yours.

In Health,

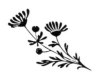

wild & well Rx

Dani Williamson, MSN, FNP

℞   Patient Name: ....

          Age: ....   Date: ....

1. Be grateful daily for things both aloud and silently. Grateful people are happier, healthier, and have a better outlook on life.

2. Go volunteer. Find a place that needs you and show up and see what happens! You will be amazed at how God shows up and shows out for those who help others.

3. Cultivate community. Start a cookout, a wine tasting, a Zoom meetup, a hike, a virtual book club… whatever it takes to get people together.

4. Guard your heart and know that even Jesus had an inner circle. Cultivate yours and keep those relationships close.

5. Cut out the soul suckers. You don't want "yes" people, but you need people that will not suck the life out of you.

6. Give yourself permission to say no and to cut ties with anyone, anything, or any activity that doesn't lift you up.

7. Set your boundaries with people and stick to them. It won't go over well at first, but your life will be more peaceful.

8. Put God first, your spouse second, and your children third… in that order!

endnotes

[1] Wekerle, H. (2016). The gut-brain connection: triggering of brain autoimmune disease by commensal gut bacteria. *Rheumatology, 55*(suppl_2), ii68–ii75.

[2] Ventura, A.; Neri, E.; Ughi, C.; Leopaldi, A.; Città, A.; & Not, T. (2000). Gluten-dependent diabetes-related and thyroid-related autoantibodies in patients with celiac disease. *The Journal of Pediatrics, 137*(2), 263–265.

[3] Poplawski, M. M.; Mastaitis, J. W.; Isoda, F.; Grosjean, F.; Zheng, F.; & Mobbs, C. V. (2011). Reversal of diabetic nephropathy by a ketogenic diet. *PloS One, 6*(4), e18604.

[4] Paterniti, S.; Dufouil, C.; & Alpérovitch, A. (2002). Long-term benzodiazepine use and cognitive decline in the elderly: the Epidemiology of Vascular Aging Study. *Journal of Clinical Psychopharmacology, 22*(3), 285–293

[5] Barker, D. J. (1998). In utero programming of chronic disease. *Clinical Science, 95*(2), 115–128.

[6] Burt, T. D. (2013). Fetal regulatory T cells and peripheral immune tolerance in utero: implications for development and disease. *American Journal of Reproductive Immunology, 69*(4), 346–358.

[7] Srivastava, S.; D'Souza, S. E.; Sen, U.; & States, J. C. (2007). In utero arsenic exposure induces early onset of atherosclerosis in ApoE−/− mice. *Reproductive Toxicology, 23*(3), 449–456.

[8] Hadley, S. K.; & Gaarder, S. M. (2005). Treatment of irritable bowel syndrome. *American Family Physician, 72*(12).

[9] Woelfel, J. A. (2004). Proton pump inhibitors associated with increased risk of Clostridium difficile diarrhea. *Pharmacist's Letter & Prescriber's Letter, 20*(8), 1.

[10] Nerandzic, M. M.; Pultz, M. J.; & Donskey, C. J. (2009). Examination of potential mechanisms to explain the association between proton pump

inhibitors and Clostridium difficile infection. *Antimicrobial Agents and Chemotherapy, 53*(10), 4133–4137.

[11] Wong H. (2015). Long-term use of diphenhydramine. *CMAJ : Canadian Medical Association Journal = Journal de l'Association Medicale Canadienne, 187*(14), 1078. doi:10.1503/cmaj.1150066

[12] Gray, S. L.; Anderson, M. L.; Dublin, S.; Hanlon, J. T.; Hubbard, R.; Walker, R.; ... & Larson, E. B. (2015). Cumulative use of strong anticholinergics and incident dementia: a prospective cohort study. *JAMA Internal Medicine, 175*(3), 401–407.

[13] Merz, B. (2015). Common anticholinergic drugs like Benadryl linked to increased dementia risk. *Cambridge (MA): Harvard Health Blog.*

[14] O'Sullivan, R. L.; Lipper, G.; & Lerner, E. A. (1998). The neuro-immuno-cutaneous-endocrine network: relationship of mind and skin. *Archives of Dermatology, 134*(11), 1431–1435.

[15] O'Neill, C. A.; Monteleone, G.; McLaughlin, J. T.; & Paus, R. (2016). The gut-skin axis in health and disease: A paradigm with therapeutic implications. *BioEssays, 38*(11), 1167–1176

[16] Bowe, W.; Patel, N. B.; & Logan, A. C. (2013). Acne vulgaris, probiotics and the gut-brain-skin axis: from anecdote to translational medicine. *Beneficial Microbes, 5*(2), 185–199.

[17] Erdman, S. E.; & Poutahidis, T. (2014). Probiotic 'glow of health': it's more than skin deep. *Beneficial Microbes, 5*(2), 109–119.

[18] Arck, P.; Handjiski, B.; Hagen, E.; Pincus, M.; Bruenahl, C.; Bienenstock, J.; & Paus, R. (2010). Is there a 'gut–brain–skin axis'?. *Experimental Dermatology, 19*(5), 401–405.

[19] Bowe, W. P.; & Logan, A. C. (2011). Acne vulgaris, probiotics and the gut-brain-skin axis-back to the future?. *Gut Pathogens, 3*(1), 1.

[20] Nesi, T. (2008). *Poison pills: the untold story of the Vioxx drug scandal.* Macmillan.

[21] Faunce, T. A. (2010). The Vioxx Pharmaceutical Scandal: Peterson v. Merke Sharpe & Dohme (Aust) Pty Ltd (2010) 184 Fcr 1. *Journal of Law and Medicine, 18*, 38–49.

[22] Ornish, D.; Scherwitz, L. W.; Billings, J. H.; Gould, K. L.; Merritt, T. A.; Sparler, S.; ... & Brand, R. J. (1998). Intensive lifestyle changes for reversal of coronary heart disease. *Jama, 280*(23), 2001–2007.

[23] Balagopal, P.; George, D.; Yarandi, H.; Funanage, V.; & Bayne, E. (2005). Reversal of obesity-related hypoadiponectinemia by lifestyle intervention: a controlled, randomized study in obese adolescents. *The Journal of Clinical Endocrinology & Metabolism, 90*(11), 6192–6197.

[24] Parekh, P. I.; Petro, A. E.; Tiller, J. M.; Feinglos, M. N.; & Surwit, R. S. (1998). Reversal of diet-induced obesity and diabetes in C57BL/6J mice. *Metabolism, 47*(9), 1089–1096.

[25] Wolffe, A. P.; & Matzke, M. A. (1999). Epigenetics: regulation through repression. *Science, 286*(5439), 481–486.

[26] Bollati, V.; & Baccarelli, A. (2010). Environmental epigenetics. *Heredity, 105*(1), 105.

[27] Esteller, M. (2008). Epigenetics in cancer. *New England Journal of Medicine, 358*(11), 1148–1159.

[28] Goldberg, A. D.; Allis, C. D.; & Bernstein, E. (2007). Epigenetics: a landscape takes shape. *Cell, 128*(4), 635–638.

[29] Stiles, J. (2011). Brain development and the nature versus nurture debate. In *Progress in Brain Research*, 189, 3–22. Elsevier.

[30] Cohen, L. J. (2018). Nature and nurture shape the microbiome. *Science Translational Medicine, 10*(449), eaau1974.

[31] Centers for Disease Control and Prevention (2019). Preventing Adverse Childhood Experiences: Leveraging the Best Available Evidence. Atlanta, GA: National Center for Injury Prevention and Control, Centers for Disease Control and Prevention.

[32] Felitti, V. J.; Anda, R. F.; Nordenberg, D.; Williamson, D. F.; Spitz, A. M.; Edwards, V.; … & Marks, J. S. (2019). Relationship of childhood abuse and household dysfunction to many of the leading causes of death in adults: The Adverse Childhood Experiences (ACE) Study. *American Journal of Preventive Medicine, 56*(6), 774–786.

[33] McEwen, B. S. (2017). Neurobiological and systemic effects of chronic stress. *Chronic Stress, 1*, 2470547017692328.

[34] Felitti, V.J.; Anda, R.F.; Nordenberg, D.; Williamson, D.F.; Spitz, A.M.; Edwards, V.; Koss, M.P.; & Marks, J.S. (1998). Relationship of childhood abuse and household dysfunction to many of the leading causes of death in adults: the adverse childhood experiences (ACE) study. *American Journal of Preventive Medicine,14*, 245–258.

[35] Bethell, C.; Gombojav, N.; Solloway, M.; & Wissow, L. (Apr 2015). Adverse Childhood Experiences, Resilience, and Mindfulness-Based Approaches: Common Denominator Issues for Children with Emotional, Mental, or Behavioral Problems. *Child and Adolescent Psychiatric Clinics of North America, 25*(2), 139–56. doi: 10.1016/j.chc.2015.12.001. Epub 2016 Jan 11.

[36] Shonkoff, J. & Gardner, A. (2012). The lifelong effects of early childhood adversity and toxic stress. *Pediatrics, 129*, e232.

[37] Van der Kolk, BA. (2014). *The Body Keeps the Score: Brain, Mind, and Body in the Healing of Trauma*. Penguin Random House, New York, NY. 10014. ISSN: 978-0-670-/8593-3.

[38] Barile, J. P.; Edwards, V. J.; Dhingra, S. S.; & Thompson, W. W. (2015). Associations among county-level social determinants of health, child maltreatment, and emotional support on health-related quality of life in adulthood. *Psychology of Violence, 5*(2), 183.

[39] Corso, P. S.; Edwards, V. J.; Fang, X.; & Mercy, J. A. (2008). Health-related quality of life among adults who experienced maltreatment during childhood. *American Journal of Public Health, 98*(6), 1094–1100.

[40] Dube, S. R.; Fairweather, D.; Pearson, W. S.; Felitti, V. J.; Anda, R. F.; & Croft, J. B. (2009). Cumulative childhood stress and autoimmune diseases in adults. *Psychosomatic Medicine, 71*(2), 243.

[41] Ports, K. A.; Holman, D. M.; Guinn, A. S.; Pampati, S.; Dyer, K. E.; Merrick, M. T.; ... & Metzler, M. (2019). Adverse childhood experiences and the presence of cancer risk factors in adulthood: a scoping review of the literature from 2005 to 2015. *Journal of Pediatric Nursing, 44*, 81–96.

[42] Holman, D. M.; Ports, K. A.; Buchanan, N. D.; Hawkins, N. A.; Merrick, M. T.; Metzler, M.; & Trivers, K. F. (2016). The association between adverse childhood experiences and risk of cancer in adulthood: a systematic review of the literature. *Pediatrics, 138*(Supplement 1), S81–S91.

[43] Brown, M. J.; Thacker, L. R.; & Cohen, S. A. (2013). Association between adverse childhood experiences and diagnosis of cancer. *PloS One, 8*(6), e65524.

[44] Brown, D. W.; Anda, R. F.; Felitti, V. J.; Edwards, V. J.; Malarcher, A. M.; Croft, J. B.; & Giles, W. H. (2010). Adverse childhood experiences are associated with the risk of lung cancer: a prospective cohort study. *BMC Public Health, 10*(1), 20.

[45] Cunningham, T. J.; Ford, E. S.; Croft, J. B.; Merrick, M. T.; Rolle, I. V.; & Giles, W. H. (2014). Sex-specific relationships between adverse childhood experiences and chronic obstructive pulmonary disease in five states. *International Journal of Chronic Obstructive Pulmonary Disease, 9*, 1033.

[46] Anda, R.; Tietjen, G.; Schulman, E.; Felitti, V.; & Croft, J. (2010). Adverse childhood experiences and frequent headaches in adults. *Headache: The Journal of Head and Face Pain, 50*(9), 1473–1481.

[47] Dong, M.; Giles, W. H.; Felitti, V. J.; Dube, S. R.; Williams, J. E., Chapman, D. P.; & Anda, R. F. (2004). Insights into causal pathways for ischemic heart disease: adverse childhood experiences study. *Circulation, 110*(13), 1761–1766.

[48] Dong, M.; Dube, S. R.; Felitti, V. J.; Giles, W. H.; & Anda, R. F. (2003). Adverse childhood experiences and self-reported liver disease: new insights into the causal pathway. *Archives of Internal Medicine, 163*(16), 1949–1956.

[49] Remigio-Baker, R. A.; Hayes, D. K.; & Reyes-Salvail, F. (2014). Adverse childhood events and current depressive symptoms among women in Hawaii: 2010 BRFSS, Hawaii. *Maternal and Child Health Journal, 18*(10), 2300–2308.

[50] Edwards, V. J.; Holden, G. W.; Felitti, V. J.; & Anda, R. F. (2003). Relationship between multiple forms of childhood maltreatment and adult mental health in community respondents: results from the adverse childhood experiences study. *American Journal of Psychiatry, 160*(8), 1453–1460.

51 Von Cheong, E.; Sinnott, C.; Dahly, D.; & Kearney, P. M. (2017). Adverse childhood experiences (ACEs) and later-life depression: perceived social support as a potential protective factor. *BMJ Open, 7*(9), e013228.

52 Chapman, D. P.; Whitfield, C. L.; Felitti, V. J.; Dube, S. R.; Edwards, V. J.; & Anda, R. F. (2004). Adverse childhood experiences and the risk of depressive disorders in adulthood. *Journal of Affective Disorders, 82*(2), 217–225.

53 Dube, S. R.; Anda, R. F.; Felitti, V. J.; Chapman, D. P.; Williamson, D. F.; & Giles, W. H. (2001). Childhood abuse, household dysfunction, and the risk of attempted suicide throughout the life span: findings from the Adverse Childhood Experiences Study. *Jama, 286*(24), 3089–3096.

54 Williamson, D. F.; Thompson, T. J.; Anda, R. F.; Dietz, W. H.; & Felitti, V. (2002). Bodyweight and obesity in adults and self-reported abuse in childhood. *International Journal of Obesity, 26*(8), 1075.

55 Anda, R. F.; Whitfield, C. L.; Felitti, V. J.; Chapman, D.; Edwards, V. J.; Dube, S. R.; & Williamson, D. F. (2002). Adverse childhood experiences, alcoholic parents, and later risk of alcoholism and depression. *Psychiatric Services, 53*(8), 1001–1009.

56 Dube, S. R.; Anda, R. F.; Felitti, V. J.; Croft, J. B.; Edwards, V. J.; & Giles, W. H. (2001). Growing up with parental alcohol abuse: exposure to childhood abuse, neglect, and household dysfunction. *Child Abuse & Neglect, 25*(12), 1627–1640.

57 Strine, T. W.; Edwards, V. J.; Dube, S. R.; Wagenfeld, M.; Dhingra, S.; Prehn, A. W.; … & Croft, J. B. (2012). The mediating sex-specific effect of psychological distress on the relationship between adverse childhood experiences and current smoking among adults. *Substance Abuse Treatment, Prevention, and Policy, 7*(1), 30.

58 Anda, R. F.; Brown, D. W.; Felitti, V. J.; Dube, S. R.; & Giles, W. H. (2008). Adverse childhood experiences and prescription drug use in a cohort study of adult HMO patients. *BMC Public Health, 8*(1), 198.

59 Dube, S. R.; Felitti, V. J.; Dong, M.; Chapman, D. P.; Giles, W. H.; & Anda, R. F. (2003). Childhood abuse, neglect, and household dysfunction and the risk of illicit drug use: the adverse childhood experiences study. *Pediatrics, 111*(3), 564–572.

60 Metzler, M.; Merrick, M. T.; Klevens, J.; Ports, K. A.; & Ford, D. C. (2017). Adverse childhood experiences and life opportunities: shifting the narrative. *Children and Youth Services Review, 72*, 141–149.

61 Brown, D. W.; Anda, R. F.; Tiemeier, H.; Felitti, V. J.; Edwards, V. J.; Croft, J. B.; & Giles, W. H. (2009). Adverse childhood experiences and the risk of premature mortality. *American Journal of Preventive Medicine, 37*(5), 389–396.

62 Anda, R. F.; Fleisher, V. I.; Felitti, V. J.; Edwards, V. J.; Whitfield, C. L.; Dube, S. R.; & Williamson, D. F. (2004). Childhood abuse, household dysfunction, and indicators of impaired adult worker performance. *The Permanente Journal, 8*(1), 30.

63 Hillis, S. D.; Anda, R. F.; Dube, S. R.; Felitti, V. J.; Marchbanks, P. A.; & Marks, J. S. (2004). The association between adverse childhood experiences and adolescent pregnancy, long-term psychosocial consequences, and fetal death. *Pediatrics, 113*(2), 320–327.

64 Hillis, S. D.; Anda, R. F.; Felitti, V. J.; & Marchbanks, P. A. (2001). Adverse childhood experiences and sexual risk behaviors in women: a retrospective cohort study. *Family Planning Perspectives*, 206–211.

65 Hillis, S. D.; Anda, R. F.; Felitti, V. J.; Nordenberg, D.; & Marchbanks, P. A. (2000). Adverse childhood experiences and sexually transmitted diseases in men and women: a retrospective study. *Pediatrics, 106*(1), e11–e11.

66 Dietz, P. M.; Spitz, A. M.; Anda, R. F.; Williamson, D. F.; McMahon, P. M.; Santelli, J. S.; … & Kendrick, J. S. (1999). Unintended pregnancy among adult women exposed to abuse or household dysfunction during their childhood. *Jama, 282*(14), 1359–1364.

67 A., V. der K. B. (2015). *The Body Keeps the Score: Mind, Brain, and Body in the Transformation of Trauma*. London: Penguin Books.

68 Middlebrooks, J. S. (2007). *The effects of childhood stress on health across the lifespan*. US Department of Health and Human Services, Centers for Disease Control and Prevention, National Center for Injury Prevention and Control.

69 Rutherford, Adam. (19 Jul 2015). Beware the pseudo gene genies. *The Guardian*.

70 Haggarty, P. (2013). Epigenetic consequences of a changing human diet. *Proceedings of the Nutrition Society, 72*(4), 363–371.

71 Pal, S.; & Tyler, J. K. (2016). Epigenetics and aging. *Science Advances, 2*(7), e1600584.

72 Tollefsbol, T. O. (2011). Epigenetics: The new science of genetics. *Handbook of Epigenetics*, 1–6. Academic Press.

73 Jaenisch, R.; & Bird, A. (2003). Epigenetic regulation of gene expression: how the genome integrates intrinsic and environmental signals. *Nature Genetics, 33*(3s), 245.

74 Merzenich, Michael M. (2013).*Soft-Wired:How the New Science of Brain Plasticity can Change Your Life*. San Francisco: Parnassus.

75 Davidson, R. J.; & Lutz, A. (2008). Buddha's Brain: Neuroplasticity and Meditation [in the spotlight]. *IEEE Signal Processing Magazine, 25*(1), 176–174.

76 Claro, S.; Paunesku, D.; & Dweck, C. S. (2016). Growth mindset tempers the effects of poverty on academic achievement. *Proceedings of the National Academy of Sciences, 113*(31), 8664–8668.

77 Dweck, C. S. (2016). *Mindset: The New Psychology of Success*. New York: Ballantine.

78 Murphy, L.; & Thomas, L. (Jun 2008). Dangers of a fixed mindset: implications of self-theories research for computer science education. *ACM SIGCSE Bulletin, 40*(3), 271–275. ACM.

79 Libby, P. (2007). Inflammatory mechanisms: the molecular basis of inflammation and disease. *Nutrition Reviews, 65*(suppl_3), S140–S146.

80 Pawelec, G.; Goldeck, D.; & Derhovanessian, E. (2014). Inflammation, ageing, and chronic disease. *Current Opinion in Immunology, 29*, 23–28.

81 Tracy, R. P. (2003). Emerging relationships of inflammation, cardiovascular disease, and chronic diseases of aging. *International Journal of Obesity, 27*(S3), S29.

82 Leonard, B. E. (2007). Inflammation, depression, and dementia: are they connected? *Neurochemical Research, 32*(10), 1749–1756.

83 Shacter, E.; & Weitzman, S. A. (2002). Chronic inflammation and cancer.

84 Figueroa-Vega, N.; Alfonso-Perez, M.; Benedicto, I.; Sanchez-Madrid, F.; Gonzalez-Amaro, R.; & Marazuela, M. (2010). Increased circulating pro-inflammatory cytokines and Th17 lymphocytes in Hashimoto's thyroiditis. *The Journal of Clinical Endocrinology & Metabolism, 95*(2), 953–962.

85 Muñoz, L. E.; Janko, C.; Schulze, C.; Schorn, C.; Sarter, K.; Schett, G.; & Herrmann, M. (2010). Autoimmunity and chronic inflammation—two clearance-related steps in the etiopathogenesis of SLE. *Autoimmunity Reviews, 10*(1), 38–42.

86 Berger, A. (2000). Th1 and Th2 responses: what are they?. *BMJ, 321*(7258), 424.

87 Cerami, A. (1992). Inflammatory cytokines. *Clinical Immunology and Immunopathology, 62*(1), S3–S10.

88 Zhang, J. M.; & An, J. (2007). Cytokines, inflammation, and pain. *International Anesthesiology Clinics, 45*(2), 27–37. doi:10.1097/AIA.0b013e318034194e

89 Vingerhoets, A. J. J. M.; & Perski, A. (2000). The psychobiology of stress. *Psychology in Medicine. Bohn Stafleu Van Loghum, Houten/Diegem*, 34–49.

90 Elenkov, I. J.; & Chrousos, G. P. (1999). Stress hormones, Th1/Th2 patterns, pro/anti-inflammatory cytokines, and susceptibility to disease. *Trends in Endocrinology & Metabolism, 10*(9), 359–368.

91 Cohen, S.; Janicki-Deverts, D.; Doyle, W. J.; Miller, G. E; Frank, E.; Rabin, B. S.; & Turner, R. B. (2012). Chronic stress, glucocorticoid receptor resistance, inflammation, and disease risk. *Proceedings of the National Academy of Sciences, 109*(16), 5995–5999.

92 Raison, C. L.; Capuron, L.; & Miller, A. H. (2006). Cytokines sing the blues: inflammation and the pathogenesis of depression. *Trends in Immunology, 27*(1), 24–31.

93 Catalán, V.; Gómez-Ambrosi, J.; Ramirez, B.; Rotellar, F.; Pastor, C.; Silva, C.; … & Frühbeck, G. (2007). Proinflammatory cytokines in obesity: impact of type 2 diabetes mellitus and gastric bypass. *Obesity Surgery, 17*(11), 1464–1474.

[94] Kim, Y. K.; Jung, H. G.; Myint, A. M.; Kim, H.; & Park, S. H. (2007). Imbalance between pro-inflammatory and anti-inflammatory cytokines in bipolar disorder. *Journal of Affective Disorders, 104*(1–3), 91–95.

[95] Raphael, I.; Nalawade, S.; Eagar, T. N.; & Forsthuber, T. G. (2015). T cell subsets and their signature cytokines in autoimmune and inflammatory diseases. *Cytokine, 74*(1), 5–17.

[96] Shan, K.; Kurrelmeyer, K.; Seta, Y.; Wang, F.; Dibbs, Z.; Deswal, A.; ... & Mann, D. L. (1997). The role of cytokines in disease progression in heart failure. *Current Opinion in Cardiology, 12*(3), 218–223.

[97] Dranoff, G. (2004). Cytokines in cancer pathogenesis and cancer therapy. *Nature Reviews Cancer, 4*(1), 11.

[98] Kemp, M. W.; Saito, M.; Nitsos, I.; Jobe, A. H.; Kallapur, S. G.; & Newnham, J. P. (2011). Exposure to in utero lipopolysaccharide induces inflammation in the fetal ovine skin. *Reproductive Sciences, 18*(1), 88–98.

[99] Campioli, E.; Martinez-Arguelles, D. B.; & Papadopoulos, V. (2014). In utero exposure to the endocrine disruptor di-(2-Ethylhexyl) phthalate promotes local adipose and systemic inflammation in adult male offspring. *Nutrition & Diabetes, 4*(5), e115.

[100] Zeng, M. Y.; Inohara, N.; & Nuñez, G. (2017). Mechanisms of inflammation-driven bacterial dysbiosis in the gut. *Mucosal Immunology, 10*(1), 18.

[101] Karin, M.; Lawrence, T.; & Nizet, V. (2006). Innate immunity gone awry: linking microbial infections to chronic inflammation and cancer. *Cell, 124*(4), 823–835.

[102] Gilden, D.; Mahalingam, R.; Nagel, M. A.; Pugazhenthi, S.; & Cohrs, R. J. (2011). The neurobiology of varicella zoster virus infection. *Neuropathology and Applied Neurobiology, 37*(5), 441–463.

[103] Pizzorno, J. E. (2018). *The Toxin Solution: How Hidden Poisons in the Air, Water, Food, and Products We Use Are Destroying Our Health and What We Can Do to Fix It*. New York: HarperOne.

[104] Kaldor, J.; Harris, J. A.; Glazer, E.; Glaser, S.; Neutra, R.; Mayberry, R.; ... & Reed, D. (1984). Statistical association between cancer incidence and major-cause mortality, and estimated residential exposure to air emissions from petroleum and chemical plants. *Environmental Health Perspectives, 54*, 319–332.

[105] Kaniwa, M. A. (2006). Preventive measures against health damage due to chemicals in household products. *Kokuritsu Iyakuhin Shokuhin Eisei Kenkyujo hokoku= Bulletin of National Institute of Health Sciences*, (124), 1–20.

[106] Patocka, J.; & Kuca, K. (2014). Irritant compounds: respiratory irritant gases. *Milit Med Sci Lett, 83*(2), 73–82.

107 Wieslander, G.; Norbäck, D.; Björnsson, E.; Janson, C.; & Boman, G. (1996). Asthma and the indoor environment: the significance of emission of formaldehyde and volatile organic compounds from newly painted indoor surfaces. *International Archives of Occupational and Environmental Health, 69*(2), 115–124.

108 Olson, W.; Vesley, D.; Bode, M.; Dubbel, P.; & Bauer, T. (1994). Hard surface cleaning performance of six alternative household cleaners under laboratory conditions. *Journal of Environmental Health*, 27–31.

109 Lee, L. K.; & Nielsen, E. G. (1987). The extent and costs of groundwater contamination by agriculture. *Journal of Soil and Water Conservation, 42*(4), 243–248.

110 Roberts, J. R.; & Karr, C. J. (2012). Pesticide exposure in children. *Pediatrics, 130*(6), e1765–e1788.

111 Cantor, K. P.; Hoover, R.; Hartge, P.; Mason, T. J.; Silverman, D. T.; Altman, R.; … & Marrett, L. D. (1987). Bladder cancer, drinking water source, and tap water consumption: a case-control study. *JNCI Journal of the National Cancer Institute, 79*(6), 1269–1279.

112 De Jongh, C. M.; Verberk, M. M.; Withagen, C. E.; Jacobs, J. J.; Rustemeyer, T.; & Kezic, S. (2006). Stratum corneum cytokines and skin irritation response to sodium lauryl sulfate. *Contact Dermatitis, 54*(6), 325–333.

113 Cohen, L.; & Jefferies, A. (2019). Environmental exposures and cancer: using the precautionary principle. *Ecancermedicalscience*.

114 Potera, C. (2011). Indoor Air Quality: Scented Products Emit a Bouquet of VOCs. *Environmental Health Perspectives, 119*(1), A16.

115 Milman, Oliver. (2019). US Cosmetics Are Full of Chemicals Banned by Europe—Why? *The Guardian*. Guardian News and Media, www.theguardian.com/us-news/2019/may/22/chemicals-in-cosmetics-us-restricted-eu.

116 Montebugnoli, L.; Servidio, D.; Miaton, R. A.; Prati, C.; Tricoci, P.; & Melloni, C. (2004). Poor oral health is associated with coronary heart disease and elevated systemic inflammatory and haemostatic factors. *Journal of Clinical Periodontology, 31*(1), 25–29.

117 Berg, A. H.; & Scherer, P. E. (2005). Adipose tissue, inflammation, and cardiovascular disease. *Circulation Research, 96*(9), 939–949.

118 Wisse, B. E. (2004). The inflammatory syndrome: the role of adipose tissue cytokines in metabolic disorders linked to obesity. *Journal of the American Society of Nephrology, 15*(11), 2792–2800.

119 Tilg, H.; & Moschen, A. R. (2006). Adipocytokines: mediators linking adipose tissue, inflammation, and immunity. *Nature Reviews Immunology, 6*(10), 772.

120 Monroe, S.; & Polk, R. (2000). Antimicrobial use and bacterial resistance. *Current Opinion in Microbiology, 3*(5), 496–501.

[121] Mellon, M.; Benbrook, C.; & Benbrook, K. L. (7 Apr 2004). Hogging It! Estimates of Antimicrobial Abuse in Livestock. *Union of Concerned Scientists*. Web.

[122] Roy, J. R.; Chakraborty, S.; & Chakraborty, T. R. (2009). Estrogen-like endocrine disrupting chemicals affecting puberty in humans--a review. *Medical Science Monitor, 15*(6), RA137–RA145.

[123] Kumar, V. S.; Rajan, C.; Divya, P.; & Sasikumar, S. (2018). Adverse effects on consumer's health caused by hormones administered in cattle. *International Food Research Journal, 25*(1).

[124] Angulo, F. J.; Baker, N. L.; Olsen, S. J.; Anderson, A.; & Barrett, T. J. (Apr 2004). Antimicrobial use in agriculture: controlling the transfer of antimicrobial resistance to humans. *Seminars in Pediatric Infectious Diseases, 159*(2), 8–85. WB Saunders.

[125] Riddell, R. H.; Tanaka, M.; & Mazzoleni, G. (1992). Non-steroidal anti-inflammatory drugs as a possible cause of collagenous colitis: a case-control study. *Gut, 33*(5), 683–686.

[126] Kaufmann, H. J.; & Taubin, H. L. (1987). Nonsteroidal anti-inflammatory drugs activate quiescent inflammatory bowel disease. *Annals of Internal Medicine, 107*(4), 513–516.

[127] Alic, M. (2000). Epidemiology supports oral contraceptives as a risk factor in Crohn's disease. *Gut, 46*(1), 140–140.

[128] Brinton, L. A.; Brogan, D. R.; Coates, R. J.; Swanson, C. A.; Potischman, N.; & Stanford, J. L. (2018). Breast cancer risk among women under 55 years of age by joint effects of usage of oral contraceptives and hormone replacement therapy. *Menopause, 25*(11), 1195–1200.

[129] Ortiz-Guerrero, G.; Amador-Muñoz, D.; Calderón-Ospina, C. A.; López-Fuentes, D.; Mesa, N.; & Orlando, M. (2018). Proton pump inhibitors and dementia: Physiopathological mechanisms and clinical consequences. *Neural Plasticity*.

[130] (2017). *Principles of Functional Medicine*. The Institute for Functional Medicine. Web.

[131] Schilling, R. (2017). Dementia And Strokes From Diet Drinks. *Dementia*.

[132] Barberger-Gateau, P.; Raffaitin, C.; Letenneur, L.; Berr, C.; Tzourio, C.; Dartigues, J. F.; & Alpérovitch, A. (2007). Dietary patterns and risk of dementia: the Three-City cohort study. *Neurology, 69*(20), 1921–1930.

[133] Ott, A.; Slooter, A. J. C.; Hofman, A.; van Harskamp, F.; Witteman, J. C. M.; Van Broeckhoven, C.; ... & Breteler, M. M. B. (1998). Smoking and risk of dementia and Alzheimer's disease in a population-based cohort study: the Rotterdam Study. *The Lancet, 351*(9119), 1840–1843.

[134] Ahlskog, J. E.; Geda, Y. E.; Graff-Radford, N. R.; & Petersen, R. C. (Sept 2011). Physical exercise as a preventive or disease-modifying treatment of dementia and brain aging. *Mayo Clinic Proceedings, 86*(9), 876–884. Elsevier.

135 Chen, J. C.; Espeland, M. A.; Brunner, R. L.; Lovato, L. C.; Wallace, R. B.; Leng, X.; ... & Manson, J. E. (2016). Sleep duration, cognitive decline, and dementia risk in older women. *Alzheimer's & Dementia, 12*(1), 21–33.

136 Lupkin, S. (27 Apr 2015). Women Put an Average of 168 Chemicals on Their Bodies Each Day, Consumer Group Says. *ABC News*. Retrieved from https://abcnews.go.com/Health/women-put-average-168-chemicals-bodies-day-consumer/story?id=30615324

137 Thongprayoon, C.; Kaewput, W.; Hatch, S. T.; Bathini, T.; Sharma, K.; Wijarnpreecha, K.; ... & Cheungpasitporn, W. (2019). Effects of probiotics on inflammation and uremic toxins among patients on dialysis: a systematic review and meta-analysis. *Digestive Diseases and Sciences, 64*(2), 469–479.

138 Dini-Andreote, F.; & van Elsas, J. D. (2019). 3 The Soil Microbiome—. *Modern Soil Microbiology, 37.*

139 Innes, J. K.; & Calder, P. C. (2018). Omega-6 fatty acids and inflammation. *Prostaglandins, Leukotrienes, and Essential Fatty Acids, 132*, 41–48.

140 Manson, J. E.; Cook, N. R.; Lee, I. M.; Christen, W.; Bassuk, S. S.; Mora, S.; ... & Friedenberg, G. (2019). Vitamin D supplements and prevention of cancer and cardiovascular disease. *New England Journal of Medicine, 380*(1), 33–44.

141 Rovoli, M.; Pappas, I.; Lalas, S.; Gortzi, O.; & Kontopidis, G. (2019). In vitro and in vivo assessment of vitamin A encapsulation in a liposome–protein delivery system. *Journal of Liposome Research, 29*(2), 142–152.

142 Noroozi, S.; Khadem Haghighian, H.; Abbasi, M.; Javadi, M.; & Goodarzi, S. (2018). A review of the therapeutic effects of frankincense. *J Qazvin Univ Med Sci 2018, 22*(1), 70–81.

143 Cardia, G. F. E.; Silva-Filho, S. E.; Silva, E. L.; Uchida, N. S.; Cavalcante, H. A. O.; Cassarotti, L. L.; ... & Cuman, R. K. N. (2018). Effect of lavender (Lavandula angustifolia) essential oil on acute inflammatory response. *Evidence-Based Complementary and Alternative Medicine*, 2018.

144 Drion, C. M.; van Scheppingen, J.; Arena, A.; Geijtenbeek, K. W.; Kooijman, L.; van Vliet, E. A.; ... & Gorter, J. A. (2018). Effects of rapamycin and curcumin on inflammation and oxidative stress in vitro and in vivo—in search of potential anti-epileptogenic strategies for temporal lobe epilepsy. *Journal of Neuroinflammation, 15*(1), 212.

145 Teitelbaum, J. (2019). A Hemp oil, CBD, and Marijuana Primer: Powerful Pain, Insomnia, and Anxiety-relieving Tools! *Alternative Therapies, 25*(S2), 221.

146 Braun, M.; Khan, Z. T.; Khan, M. B.; Kumar, M.; Ward, A.; Achyut, B. R.; ... & Dhandapani, K. M. (2018). Selective activation of cannabinoid receptor-2 reduces neuroinflammation after traumatic brain injury via alternative macrophage polarization. *Brain, Behavior, and Immunity, 68*, 224–237.

[147] Christopher, G.; Fleming, D.; Harris, R.; Spencer, T.; Gibson, S. M.; & Harris, C. (2018). *State of Obesity: Better Policies for a Healthier America*. Princeton (NJ): Robert Wood Johnson Foundation.

[148] Bourgeois, J. (2018). Identifying and Predicting Areas of Increasing Heart Disease Mortality in the United States.

[149] Schoeni, R. F.; Freedman, V. A.; & Langa, K. M. (2018). Introduction to a supplement on population level trends in dementia: Causes, disparities, and projections. *The Journals of Gerontology: Series B, 73*(suppl_1), S1–S9.

[150] Centers for Disease Control and Prevention United States Cancer Statistics. Lasted updated 2016. Web

[151] Heron, M. (24 Jun 2019). Deaths: Leading Causes for 2017. *National Vital Statistics Reports 68*(6).

[152] https://www.aarda.org/news-information/statistics/

[153] https://www.medicalnewstoday.com/articles/246960.php#1

[154] https://clincalc.com/DrugStats/Top300Drugs.aspx

[155] Meade, S. J.; Reid, E. A.; & Gerrard, J. A. (2005). The impact of processing on the nutritional quality of food proteins. *Journal of AOAC International, 88*(3), 904–922.

[156] Fennema, O. R.; Damodaran, S.; & Parkin, K. L. (2017). Introduction to food chemistry. *Fennema's Food Chemistry*, 1–16. CRC Press.

[157] Choi, S. W.; Claycombe, K. J.; Martinez, J. A.; Friso, S.; & Schalinske, K. L. (2013). Nutritional epigenomics: a portal to disease prevention.

[158] Sebastiani, P.; Gurinovich, A.; Nygaard, M.; Sasaki, T.; Sweigart, B.; Bae, H.; … & Arai, Y. (2018). APOE alleles and extreme human longevity. *The Journals of Gerontology: Series A, 74*(1), 44–51.

[159] Doll, R.; & Peto, R. (1981). The causes of cancer: quantitative estimates of avoidable risks of cancer in the United States today. *JNCI: Journal of the National Cancer Institute, 66*(6), 1192–1308.

[160] Panagiotou, G.; & Nielsen, J. (2009). Nutritional systems biology: definitions and approaches. *Annual Review of Nutrition, 29*, 329–339.

[161] Suzuki, M.; Willcox, D. C.; & Willcox, B. (2015). Okinawa centenarian study: investigating healthy aging among the world's longest-lived people. *Encyclopedia of Geropsychology*, 1–5.

[162] Fraser, G. E.; & Shavlik, D. J. (2001). Ten years of life: is it a matter of choice?. *Archives of Internal Medicine, 161*(13), 1645–1652.

[163] Carolan, M. (2018). *The Real Cost of Cheap Food*. Routledge.

[164] Allen, G. J.; Albala, K.n, eds. (2007). *The Business of Food: Encyclopedia of the Food and Drink Industries*. ABC-CLIO. p. 288. ISBN 978-0-313-33725-3.

165 Trautmann, N. M.; & Porter, K. S. (2012). Modern Agriculture: Its Effects on the Environment. Pesticide Safety Education Program. Retrieved from http://psep.cce.cornell.edu/facts-slides-self/facts/mod-ag-grw85.aspx

166 Pandrangi, S.; & Laborde, L. F. (2004). Retention of folate, carotenoids, and other quality characteristics in commercially packaged fresh spinach. *Journal of Food Science, 69*(9), C702–C707.

167 Interagency Agricultural Projections Committee. (Feb 2017). *USDA Agricultural Projections to 2026.* United States Department of Agriculture. Retrieved from https://www.ers.usda.gov/webdocs/publications/82539/oce-2017-1. pdf?v=42788

168 Byrnes, S. E.; Miller, J. C.; Denyer, G. S. (Jun 1995). Amylopectin starch promotes the development of insulin resistance in rats. *Journal of Nutrition.* Pubmed: 7782895

169 Behall, K. M.; Scholfield D. J.; Yuhaniak, I.; Canary, J. (Feb 1989). Diets containing high amylose vs amylopectin starch: effects on metabolic variables in human subjects. *American Journal of Clinical Nutrition.* Pubmed: 2644803

170 (Mar 2017). *National Center for Health Statistics. Centers for Disease Control and Prevention.* Retrieved from https://www.cdc.gov/nchs/fastats/diet.htm

171 World Health Organization. (2015). Evaluation of five organophosphate insecticides and herbicides. *IARC Monographs, 112.*

172 Pavelka, S. (2004). Metabolism of bromide and its interference with the metabolism of iodine. *Physiological Research, 53,* S81–90.

173 Biosafety Clearing-House Living Modified Organism identity database. Bch. cbd.int. Retrieved 2 Jan 2020.

174 Sapone, A.; Lammers, K. M.; Casolaro, V.; Cammarota, M.; Giuliano, M. T.; De Rosa, M.; … & Esposito, P. (2011). Divergence of gut permeability and mucosal immune gene expression in two gluten-associated conditions: celiac disease and gluten sensitivity. *BMC Medicine, 9*(1), 23.

175 Sapone, A.; Bai, J. C.; Ciacci, C.; Dolinsek, J.; Green, P. H.; Hadjivassiliou, M.; … & Ullrich, R. (2012). Spectrum of gluten-related disorders: consensus on new nomenclature and classification. *BMC Medicine, 10*(1), 13.

176 Troncone, R.; & Jabri, B. (2011). Coeliac disease and gluten sensitivity. *Journal of Internal Medicine, 269*(6), 582–590.

177 Klee, W. A.; & Zioudrou, C. (1980). The possible actions of peptides with opioid activity derived from pepsin hydrolysates of wheat gluten and of other constituents of gluten in the function of the central nervous system. *Biochemistry of Schizophrenia and Addiction*, 53–76. Springer, Dordrecht.

178 Bressan, P.; & Kramer, P. (2016). Bread and other edible agents of mental disease. *Frontiers in Human Neuroscience, 10,* 130.

[179] Catassi, C.; Fabiani, E.; Corrao, G.; Barbato, M.; De Renzo, A.; Carella, A. M.; ... & Bertolani, P. (2002). Risk of non-Hodgkin lymphoma in celiac disease. *Jama, 287*(11), 1413–1419.

[180] Freeman, H. J. (2009). Adult celiac disease and its malignant complications. *Gut and Liver, 3*(4), 237.

[181] Swallow, D. M. (2003). Genetics of lactase persistence and lactose intolerance. *Annual Review of Genetics, 37*(1), 197–219.

[182] Scrimshaw, N. S.; & Murray, E. B. (1988). The acceptability of milk and milk products in populations with a high prevalence of lactose intolerance. *The American Journal of Clinical Nutrition, 48*(4), 1142–1159.

[183] Szilagyi, A.; Galiatsatos, P.; & Xue, X. (2015). Systematic review and meta-analysis of lactose digestion, its impact on intolerance and nutritional effects of dairy food restriction in inflammatory bowel diseases. *Nutrition Journal, 15*(1), 67.

[184] Cumming, R. G.; & Klineberg, R. J. (1994). Case-control study of risk factors for hip fractures in the elderly. *American Journal of Epidemiology, 139*(5), 493–503.

[185] Hussain, S. M.; Cicuttini, F. M.; Giles, G. G.; Graves, S. E.; Wluka, A. E.; & Wang, Y. (2017). Association between dairy product consumption and incidence of total hip arthroplasty for osteoarthritis. *The Journal of Rheumatology, 44*(7), 1066–1070.

[186] Wu, Y.; Wu, T.; Wu, J.; Zhao, L.; Li, Q.; Varghese, Z.; ... & Ruan, X. Z. (2013). Chronic inflammation exacerbates glucose metabolism disorders in C57BL/6J mice fed with high-fat diet. *Journal of Endocrinology, 219*(3), 195–204.

[187] Knoflach, P.; Park, B. H.; Cunningham, R.; Weiser, M. M.; & Albini, B. (1987). Serum antibodies to cow's milk proteins in ulcerative colitis and Crohn's disease. *Gastroenterology, 92*(2), 479–485.

[188] Truswell, A. S. (2005). The A2 milk case: a critical review. *European Journal of Clinical Nutrition, 59*(5), 623.

[189] He, M.; Sun, J.; Jiang, Z. Q.; & Yang, Y. X. (2017). Effects of cow's milk beta-casein variants on symptoms of milk intolerance in Chinese adults: a multicentre, randomized controlled study. *Nutrition Journal, 16*(1), 72.

[190] Sermet, M. O. (2019). *Investigation of the Acute Digestive Symptoms Caused by Milks with Different Beta-casein Protein Variants in Dairy Intolerant Persons.* (Doctoral dissertation, figshare).

[191] Defilippi, C.; Gomez, E.; Charlin, V.; & Silva, C. (1995). Inhibition of small intestinal motility by casein: a role of beta casomorphins?. *Nutrition, 11*(6), 751–754. Burbank, Los Angeles County, Calif.

[192] He, M.; Sun, J.; Jiang, Z. Q.; & Yang, Y. X. (2017). Effects of cow's milk beta-casein variants on symptoms of milk intolerance in Chinese adults: a multicentre, randomised controlled study. *Nutrition Journal, 16*(1), 72.

[193] Jianqin, S.; Leiming, X.; Lu, X.; Yelland, G. W.; Ni, J.; & Clarke, A. J. (2015). Effects of milk containing only A2 beta-casein versus milk containing both A1 and A2 beta-casein proteins on gastrointestinal physiology, symptoms of discomfort, and cognitive behavior of people with self-reported intolerance to traditional cows' milk. *Nutrition Journal, 15*(1), 35.

[194] Melnik, B. C. (2009). Milk–the promoter of chronic Western diseases. *Medical Hypotheses, 72*(6), 631–639.

[195] Melnik, B. C. (2011). Evidence for acne-promoting effects of milk and other insulinotropic dairy products. *Milk and Milk Products in Human Nutrition, 67,* 131–145. Karger Publishers.

[196] Kaaks, R. (2004, November). Nutrition, insulin, IGF-1 metabolism, and cancer risk: a summary of epidemiological evidence. *Novartis Foundation Symposium*, 247–264. Chichester; New York; John Wiley; 1999.

[197] Bordoni, A.; Danesi, F.; Dardevet, D.; Dupont, D.; Fernandez, A. S.; Gille, D.; ... & Shahar, D. R. (2017). Dairy products and inflammation: a review of the clinical evidence. *Critical Reviews in Food Science and Nutrition, 57*(12), 2497–2525.

[198] Mace, K.; Aguilar, F.; Wang, J. S.; Vautravers, P.; Gomez-Lechon, M.; Gonzalez, F. J.; ... & Pfeifer, A. M. (1997). Aflatoxin B1-induced DNA adduct formation and p53 mutations in CYP450-expressing human liver cell lines. *Carcinogenesis, 18*(7), 1291–1297.

[199] https://www.foxnews.com/health/aflatoxin-an-invisible-food-hazard

[200] Ardekani, A. M.; & Shirzad, M. (2019). Genetically Modified (GM) foods and the risk to human health and environment.

[201] Parker, K.; Salas, M.; & Nwosu, V. C. (2010). High-fructose corn syrup: Production, Uses and Public Health Concern. *Biotechnology and Molecular Biology Review*. Retrieved from http://www.academicjournals.org/article/article1380113250_Parker%20et%20al.pdf

[202] Stanhope, K. L. (2016). Sugar consumption, metabolic disease and obesity: The state of the controversy. *Critical Reviews in Clinical Laboratory Sciences, 53*(1), 52–67.

[203] Ruanpeng, D.; Thongprayoon, C.; Cheungpasitporn, W.; & Harindhanavudhi, T. (2017). Sugar and artificially sweetened beverages linked to obesity: a systematic review and meta-analysis. *QJM: An International Journal of Medicine, 110*(8), 513–520.

[204] Yang, Q.; Zhang, Z.; Gregg, E. W.; Flanders, W. D.; Merritt, R.; & Hu, F. B. (2014). Added sugar intake and cardiovascular diseases mortality among US adults. *JAMA Internal Medicine, 174*(4), 516–524.

[205] Thayer, Robert E. (Jan 1987). Energy, tiredness, and tension effects of a sugar snack versus moderate exercise. *Journal of Personality and Social Psychology, 52*(1), 119–125.

[206] World Health Organization. (2003). Controlling the global obesity epidemic.

[207] Yudkin, J. (1967). Evolutionary and historical changes in dietary carbohydrates. *The American Journal of Clinical Nutrition, 20*(2), 108–115.

[208] DiNicolantonio, J. J.; O'Keefe, J. H.; & Wilson, W. L. (2018). Sugar addiction: is it real? A narrative review. *British Journal of Sports Medicine, 52*(14), 910–913.

[209] Aune, D. (2012). Soft drinks, aspartame, and the risk of cancer and cardiovascular disease.

[210] Fung, T. T.; Malik, V.; Rexrode, K. M.; Manson, J. E.; Willett, W. C.; & Hu, F. B. (2009). Sweetened beverage consumption and risk of coronary heart disease in women. *The American Journal of Clinical Nutrition, 89*(4), 1037–1042.

[211] Wagner-Schuman, M.; Richardson, J. R.; Auinger, P.; Braun, J. M.; Lanphear, B. P.; Epstein, J. N.; ... & Froehlich, T. E. (2015). Association of pyrethroid pesticide exposure with attention-deficit/hyperactivity disorder in a nationally representative sample of US children. *Environmental Health, 14*(1), 44.

[212] Liu, Y.; Wheaton, A. G.; Chapman D. P.; Cunningham T. J.; Lu, H.; & Croft, J. B. (2014). Prevalence of Healthy Sleep Duration among Adults — United States. MMWR Morb Mortal Wkly Rep 2016;65:137–141. DOI: http://dx.doi.org/10.15585/mmwr.mm6506a1external icon.

[213] Janszky, I.; Ahnve, S.; Ljung, R.; Mukamal, K. J.; Gautam, S.; Wallentin, L.; & Stenestrand, U. (2012). Daylight saving time shifts and incidence of acute myocardial infarction–Swedish Register of Information and Knowledge About Swedish Heart Intensive Care Admissions (RIKS-HIA). *Sleep Medicine, 13*(3), 237–242.

[214] Coren, S. (1996). Accidental death and the shift to daylight savings time. *Perceptual and Motor Skills, 83*(3), 921–922.

[215] Monk, T. H.; & Aplin, L. C. (1980). Spring and autumn daylight saving time changes: studies of adjustment in sleep timings, mood, and efficiency. *Ergonomics, 23*(2), 167–178.

[216] Billiard, M.; & Bentley, A. (2004). Is insomnia best categorized as a symptom or a disease?. *Sleep Medicine, 5*, S35–S40.

[217] Neubauer, D. N. (2004). Chronic insomnia: current issues. *Clinical Cornerstone, 6*(1), S17–S22.

[218] Johnson, E. O.; Roth, T.; & Breslau, N. (2006). The association of insomnia with anxiety disorders and depression: exploration of the direction of risk. *Journal of Psychiatric Research, 40*(8), 700–708.

[219] Stoller, M. K. (1994). Economic effects of insomnia. *Clinical Therapeutics: The International Peer-Reviewed Journal of Drug Therapy.*

[220] Li, X.; Liu, Y.; Rich, S. S.; Rotter, J. I.; Redline, S.; & Sofer, T. (2019). 0291 Sleep Disordered Breathing Associated with Epigenetic Age Acceleration: Evidence from the Multi-Ethnic Study of Atherosclerosis. *Sleep, 42*(Supplement_1), A118–A119.

[221] Tasali, E.; & Ip, M. S. (2008). Obstructive sleep apnea and metabolic syndrome: alterations in glucose metabolism and inflammation. *Proceedings of the American Thoracic Society, 5*(2), 207–217.

[222] Andrews, J. G.; & Oei, T. P. (2004). The roles of depression and anxiety in the understanding and treatment of obstructive sleep apnea syndrome. *Clinical Psychology Review, 24*(8), 1031–1049.

[223] Parish, J. M.; & Somers, V. K. (2004, August). Obstructive sleep apnea and cardiovascular disease. *Mayo Clinic Proceedings, 79*(8), 1036–1046. Elsevier.

[224] Hiestand, D. M.; Britz, P.; Goldman, M.; & Phillips, B. (2006). Prevalence of symptoms and risk of sleep apnea in the US population. *Chest, 130*(3), 780–786.

[225] Winkelman, J. W. (2006). Considering the causes of RLS. *European Journal of Neurology, 13*, 8–14.

[226] Hung, C. M.; Li, Y. C.; Chen, H. J.; Lu, K.; Liang, C. L.; Liliang, P. C.; ... & Wang, K. W. (2018). Risk of dementia in patients with primary insomnia: a nationwide population-based case-control study. *BMC Psychiatry, 18*(1), 38.

[227] Kitamura, T.; Miyazaki, S.; Sulaiman, H. B.; Akaike, R.; Ito, Y.; & Suzuki, H. (2020). Insomnia and obstructive sleep apnea as potential triggers of dementia: is personalized prediction and prevention of the pathological cascade applicable?. *EPMA Journal*, 1–11.

[228] https://alert.psychnews.org/2019/07/frequent-use-of-medications-for-sleep.html

[229] Dyer, O. (2019). FDA issues black box warnings on common insomnia drugs. *BMJ: British Medical Journal (Online)*, 365.

[230] McCarthy, A.; Wafford, K.; Shanks, E.; Ligocki, M.; Edgar, D. M.; & Dijk, D. J. (2016). REM sleep homeostasis in the absence of REM sleep: Effects of antidepressants. *Neuropharmacology, 108*, 415–425.

[231] Doufas, A. G.; Panagiotou, O. A.; Panousis, P.; Wong, S. S.; & Ioannidis, J. P. (Jan 2017). Insomnia from drug treatments: evidence from meta-analyses of randomized trials and concordance with prescribing information. *Mayo Clinic Proceedings, 92*(1), 72–87. Elsevier.

[232] Bosch, O. J.; Dabrowska, J.; Modi, M. E.; Johnson, Z. V.; Keebaugh, A. C.; Barrett, C. E.; ... & Neumann, I. D. (2016). Oxytocin in the nucleus accumbens shell reverses CRFR2-evoked passive stress-coping after partner loss in monogamous male prairie voles. *Psychoneuroendocrinology, 64*, 66–78.

[233] Lancel, M.; Krömer, S.; & Neumann, I. D. (2003). Intracerebral oxytocin modulates sleep–wake behaviour in male rats. *Regulatory Peptides, 114*(2–3), 145–152.

[234] Jain, V.; Marbach, J.; Kimbro, S.; Andrade, D. C.; Jain, A.; Capozzi, E.; ... & Mendelowitz, D. (2017). Benefits of oxytocin administration in obstructive sleep apnea. *American Journal of Physiology-Lung Cellular and Molecular Physiology, 313*(5), L825–L833.

235 Zhang, L.; Ou, X.; Zhu, T.; & Lv, X. (2019). Beneficial effects of estrogens in obstructive sleep apnea hypopnea syndrome. *Sleep and Breathing*, 1–7.

236 Kolanu, B. R.; Vadakedath, S.; Boddula, V.; & Kandi, V. (2020). Activities of Serum Magnesium and Thyroid Hormones in Pre-, Peri-, and Post-menopausal Women. *Cureus, 12*(1).

237 https://www.sleepfoundation.org/insomnia/older-adults

238 Kolla, B. P.; He, J. P.; Mansukhani, M. P.; Frye, M. A.; & Merikangas, K. (2020). Excessive sleepiness and associated symptoms in the US adult population: prevalence, correlates, and comorbidity. *Sleep Health, 6*(1), 79–87.

239 Hershner, S. (2020). Sleep and academic performance: Measuring the impact of sleep. *Current Opinion in Behavioral Sciences, 33*, 51–56.

240 Brum, M. C. B.; Dantas Filho, F. F.; Schnorr, C. C.; Bertoletti, O. A.; Bottega, G. B.; & da Costa Rodrigues, T. (2020). Night shift work, short sleep and obesity. *Diabetology & Metabolic Syndrome, 12*(1), 13.

241 Van der Lely, S.; Frey, S.; Garbazza, C.; Wirz-Justice, A.; Jenni, O. G.; Steiner, R.; … & Schmidt, C. (2015). Blue blocker glasses as a countermeasure for alerting effects of evening light-emitting diode screen exposure in male teenagers. *Journal of Adolescent Health, 56*(1), 113–119.

242 Burman, O.; Marsella, G.; Di Clemente, A.; & Cervo, L. (2018). The effect of exposure to low frequency electromagnetic fields (EMF) as an integral part of the housing system on anxiety-related behaviour, cognition and welfare in two strains of laboratory mouse. *Plos One, 13*(5), e0197054.

243 Carpenter, D. O. (2019). Extremely low frequency electromagnetic fields and cancer: How source of funding affects results. *Environmental Research, 178*, 108688.

244 Bagheri Hosseinabadi, M.; Khanjani, N.; Ebrahimi, M. H.; Haji, B.; & Abdolahfard, M. (2019). The effect of chronic exposure to extremely low-frequency electromagnetic fields on sleep quality, stress, depression and anxiety. *Electromagnetic Biology and Medicine, 38*(1), 96–101.

245 Rubin, G. J.; Munshi, J. D.; & Wessely, S. (2005). Electromagnetic hypersensitivity: a systematic review of provocation studies. *Psychosomatic Medicine, 67*(2), 224–232.

246 US Preventive Services Task Force: Grossman, D. C.; Bibbins-Domingo, K.; Curry, S. J.; Barry, M. J.; Davidson, K. W.; Doubeni, C. A.; Epling, J. W., Jr; Kemper, A. R.; Krist, A. H.; Kurth, A. E.; Landefeld, C. S.; Mangione, C. M.; Phipps, M. G.; Silverstein, M.; Simon, M. A.; & Tseng, C. W. (2017). Screening for Obesity in Children and Adolescents: US Preventive Services Task Force Recommendation Statement. *JAMA, 317*(23), 2417–2426. https://doi.org/10.1001/jama.2017.6803

[247] US Preventive Services Task Force, Grossman, D. C., Bibbins-Domingo, K., Curry, S. J., Barry, M. J., Davidson, K. W., Doubeni, C. A., Epling, J. W., Jr, Kemper, A. R., Krist, A. H., Kurth, A. E., Landefeld, C. S., Mangione, C. M., Phipps, M. G., Silverstein, M., Simon, M. A., & Tseng, C. W. (2017). Screening for Obesity in Children and Adolescents: US Preventive Services Task Force Recommendation Statement. JAMA, 317(23), 2417–2426. https://doi.org/10.1001/jama.2017.6803

[248] U.S. Preventive Services Task Force. (2016). Final update summary: Healthful diet and physical activity for cardiovascular disease prevention in adults without known risk factors: Behavioral counseling. Retrieved from https://www.uspreventiveservicestaskforce.org/Page/Document/UpdateSummaryFinal/healthful-diet-and-physical-activity-for-cardiovascular-disease-prevention-in-adults-without-known-risk-factors-behavioral-counseling

[249] Ward, B. W.; Clarke, T. C.; Freeman, G.; & Schiller, J. S. (2013). Early release of selected estimates based on data from the January–September 2014 National Health Interview Survey.

[250] Booth, F. W.; Roberts, C. K.; & Laye, M. J. (2011). Lack of exercise is a major cause of chronic diseases. *Comprehensive Physiology, 2*(2), 1143–1211.

[251] https://www.finder.com/unused-gym-memberships

[252] Raastad, T.; Kirketeig, A.; Wolf, D.; Paulsen, G. (Jul 2012). Powerlifters improved strength and muscular adaptations to a greater extent when equal total training volume was divided into 6 compared to 3 training sessions per week (abstract). *Book of Abstracts, 17th annual conference of the ECSS, Brugge,* 4–7.

[253] Broad, W. J. (2012). *The Science of Yoga: The Risks and the Rewards.* Simon and Schuster.

[254] Streeter, C. C.; Gerbarg, P. L.; Saper, R. B.; Ciraulo, D. A.; & Brown, R. P. (2012). Effects of yoga on the autonomic nervous system, gamma-aminobutyric-acid, and allostasis in epilepsy, depression, and post-traumatic stress disorder. *Medical Hypotheses, 78*(5), 571–579.

[255] Thomas, Jr., W. C. (1994). Exercise, age, and bones. *Southern Medical Journal, 87*(5), S23–5.

[256] Michel, B. A.; Lane, N. E.; Bloch, D. A.; Jones, H. H.; & Fries, J. F. (1991). Effect of changes in weight-bearing exercise on lumbar bone mass after age fifty. *Annals of Medicine, 23*(4), 397–401.

[257] Schwartz, R. S.; & Evans, W. J. (1995). Effects of exercise on body composition and functional capacity of the elderly. *The Journals of Gerontology Series A: Biological Sciences and Medical Sciences, 50*(Special Issue), 147–150.

[258] Hackney, M. E.; & Earhart, G. M. (2009). Effects of dance on movement control in Parkinson's disease: a comparison of Argentine tango and American ballroom. *Journal of Rehabilitation Medicine, 41*(6), 475–481.

[259] Lazarou, I.; Parastatidis, T.; Tsolaki, A.; Gkioka, M.; Karakostas, A.; Douka, S.; & Tsolaki, M. (2017). International ballroom dancing against neurodegeneration: a randomized controlled trial in Greek community-dwelling elders with mild cognitive impairment. *American Journal of Alzheimer's Disease & Other Dementias, 32*(8), 489–499.

[260] Iwayama, K.; Kurihara, R.; Nabekura, Y.; Kawabuchi, R.; Park, I.; Kobayashi, M.; ... & Tokuyama, K. (2015). Exercise increases 24-h fat oxidation only when it is performed before breakfast. *EBioMedicine, 2*(12), 2003–2009.

[261] Marshall, S. J.; Jones, D. A.; Ainsworth, B. E.; Reis, J. P.; Levy, S. S.; & Macera, C. A. (2007). Race/ethnicity, social class, and leisure-time physical inactivity. *Medicine & Science in Sports & Exercise, 39*(1), 44–51.

[262] Human Microbiome Project / Funded Research. *The NIH Common Fund*. Retrieved 9 Oct 2020.

[263] Human Microbiome Project / Program Initiatives. *The NIH Common Fund*. Retrieved 9 Oct 2020.

[264] NIH Human Microbiome Project—About the Human Microbiome. hmpdacc.org. Retrieved 9 Oct 2020.

[265] Infant Mortality | Maternal and Infant Health | Reproductive Health | CDC. www.cdc.gov. 2018-01-02. Retrieved 10 Oct 2020.

[266] Consortium, VCU, Vaginal Microbiome. *Vaginal Microbiome Consortium*. vmc.vcu.edu. Retrieved 10 Oct 2020.

[267] National Diabetes Statistics Report | Data & Statistics | Diabetes | CDC. www.cdc.gov. 2018-03-09. Retrieved 9 Oct 2020.

[268] Integrated Personal Omics Profiling | Integrated Personal Omics Profiling | Stanford Medicine. med.stanford.edu. Retrieved 10 Oct 2020.

[269] Methé, B. A.; Nelson, K. E.; Pop, M.; Creasy, H. H.; Giglio, M. G.; Huttenhower, C.; ... & Chinwalla, A. T. (2012). A framework for human microbiome research. *Nature, 486*(7402), 215.

[270] Mays, S. (2018). Micronutrient deficiency diseases: anemia, scurvy, and rickets. *The International Encyclopedia of Biological Anthropology*, 1–5.

[271] Selma-Royo, M.; Tarrazó, M.; García-Mantrana, I.; Gómez-Gallego, C.; Salminen, S.; & Collado, M. C. (2019). Shaping microbiota during the first 1000 days of life. *Probiotics and Child Gastrointestinal Health*, 3–24. Springer, Cham.

[272] Harman, T.; & Wakeford, A. (2017). *Your Baby's Microbiome: The Critical Role of Vaginal Birth and Breastfeeding for Lifelong Health*. Chelsea Green Publishing.

[273] Dahlhamer, J. M.; Zammitti, E. P.; Ward, B. W.; Wheaton, A. G.; & Croft, J. B. (2016). Prevalence of inflammatory bowel disease among adults aged 18 years— United States, 2015. *Morbidity and Mortality Weekly Report, 65*(42), 1166–1169.

274 Dahlhamer, J. M.; Zammitti, E. P.; Ward, B. W.; Wheaton, A. G.; & Croft, J. B. (2016). Prevalence of inflammatory bowel disease among adults aged 18 years—United States, 2015. *Morbidity and Mortality Weekly Report, 65*(42), 1166–1169.

275 Schnabel, L.; Buscail, C.; Sabate, J. M.; Bouchoucha, M.; Kesse-Guyot, E.; Allès, B.; … & Julia, C. (2018). Association between ultra-processed food consumption and functional gastrointestinal disorders: Results from the French NutriNet-Santé cohort. *American Journal of Gastroenterology, 113*(8), 1217–1228.

276 Gudipally, P. R.; & Sharma, G. K. (2020). Premenstrual Syndrome. *StatPearls* [Internet].

277 Wald, A.; Scarpignato, C.; Kamm, M. A; et al. The burden of constipation on quality of life: results of a multinational survey. Aliment Pharmacol Ther 2007;26:227–36.

278 Brown-Lieberson, S. (2019). Attitudes and Knowledge about Irritable Bowel Syndrome (IBS) among Family Medicine Physicians and IBS Patients.

279 Ballou, S.; McMahon, C.; Lee, H. N.; Katon, J.; Shin, A.; Rangan, V.; … & Iturrino, J. (2019). Effects of irritable bowel syndrome on daily activities vary among subtypes based on results from the IBS in America Survey. *Clinical Gastroenterology and Hepatology, 17*(12), 2471–2478.

280 https://www.crohnscolitisfoundation.org/sites/default/files/legacy/assets/pdfs/IBDoverview.pdf

281 Jandhyala, S. M.; Talukdar, R.; Subramanyam, C.; Vuyyuru, H.; Sasikala, M.; & Reddy, D. N. (2015). Role of the normal gut microbiota. *World Journal of Gastroenterology, 21*(29), 8787–8803. Retrieved from http://doi.org/10.3748/wjg.v21.i29.8787

282 Rajpoot, M.; Sharma, A. K.; Sharma, A.; & Gupta, G. K. (Oct 2018). Understanding the microbiome: emerging biomarkers for exploiting the microbiota for personalized medicine against cancer. *Seminars in Cancer Biology, 52*, 1–8. Academic Press.

283 Meadow, J. F.; Altrichter, A. E.; Bateman, A. C.; Stenson, J.; Brown, G. Z.; Green, J. L.; Bohannan, B. J. (Sept 2015). Humans differ in their personal microbial cloud. PeerJ. 3:e1258 https://doi.org/10.7717/peerj.1258

284 Slyepchenko, A.; Maes, M.; Machado-Vieira, R.; Anderson, G.; Solmi, M.; Sanz, Y.; … & Carvalho, A. F (2016). Intestinal dysbiosis, gut hyperpermeability and bacterial translocation: missing links between depression, obesity and type 2 diabetes. *Current Pharmaceutical Design, 22*(40), 6087–6106.

285 Zhuang, Z. Q.; Shen, L. L.; Li, W. W.; Fu, X.; Zeng, F.; Gui, L.; … & Zheng, P. (2018). Gut microbiota is altered in patients with Alzheimer's disease. *Journal of Alzheimer's disease, 63*(4), 1337–1346.

[286] Taams, L. S. (2019). Neuroimmune interactions: how the nervous and immune systems influence each other. *Clinical & Experimental Immunology, 197*(3), 276–277.

[287] Ren, C.; Liu, J.; Zhou, J.; Liang, H.; Wang, Y.; Sun, Y.; ... & Yin, Y. (2018). Low levels of serum serotonin and amino acids identified in migraine patients. *Biochemical and Biophysical Research Communications, 496*(2), 267–273.

[288] Gokani, T. The Prevalence of Food Allergies in Migraine Patients. Headache. Abstract 2012; 54

[289] Centers for Disease Control and Prevention. (2016). CDC: 1 in 3 antibiotic prescriptions unnecessary.

[290] Cummings, J. H.; Macfarlane, G. T.; Englyst, H. N. (Feb 2001). Prebiotic digestion and fermentation. *American Journal of Clinical Nutrition*. Pubmed, 11157351.

[291] Ghanim, H.; Abuaysheh, S.; Sia, C. L.; Korzeniewski, K.; Chaudhuri, A.; Fernandez-Real, J. M.; & Dandona, P. (2009). Increase in plasma endotoxin concentrations and the expression of Toll-like receptors and suppressor of cytokine signaling-3 in mononuclear cells after a high-fat, high-carbohydrate meal: implications for insulin resistance. *Diabetes Care, 32*(12), 2281–2287. https://doi.org/10.2337/dc09-0979

[292] Moludi, J.; Maleki, V.; Jafari-Vayghyan, H.; Vaghef-Mehrabany, E.; & Alizadeh, M. (2020). Metabolic endotoxemia and cardiovascular disease: A systematic review about potential roles of prebiotics and probiotics. *Clinical and Experimental Pharmacology and Physiology, 47*(6), 927–939.

[293] Valentin, N.; Camilleri, M.; Carlson, P.; Harrington, S. C.; Eckert, D.; O'Neill, J.; ... & Acosta, A. (2017). Potential mechanisms of effects of serum-derived bovine immunoglobulin/protein isolate therapy in patients with diarrhea-predominant irritable bowel syndrome. *Physiological Reports, 5*(5), e13170.

[294] Duggan, C.; Gannon, J.; & Walker, W. A. (2002). Protective nutrients and functional foods for the gastrointestinal tract. *The American Journal of Clinical Nutrition, 75*(5), 789–808.

[295] Raveendra, K. R.; Jayachandra, S. V.; Sushma, K. R.; Allan, J. J.; Goudar, K. S.; ... & Agarwal, A. (2012). An Extract of *Glycyrrhiza glabra* (GutGard) Alleviates Symptoms of Functional Dyspepsia: A Randomized, Double-Blind, Placebo-Controlled Study. *Evidence-Based Complementary and Alternative Medicine*: eCAM, 2012, 216970. http://doi.org/10.1155/2012/216970

[296] http://www.ncbi.nlm.nih.gov/pubmed/17420159

[297] Rezazadeh, K.; Aliashrafi, S.; Asghari-Jafarabadi, M.; & Ebrahimi-Mameghani, M. (2018). Antioxidant response to artichoke leaf extract supplementation in metabolic syndrome: A double-blind placebo-controlled randomized clinical trial. *Clinical Nutrition, 37*(3), 790–796.

[298] Aggarwal, A. (2019). *Heal Your Body, Cure Your Mind: Leaky Gut, Adrenal Fatigue,*

Liver Detox, Mental Health, Anxiety, Depression, Disease & Trauma. Mindfulness, Holistic Therapies, Nutrition & Food (Vol. 1). Dr. Ameet Aggarwal ND.

[299] Francino, M. P. (2016). Antibiotics and the human gut microbiome: dysbioses and accumulation of resistances. *Frontiers in Microbiology, 6*, 1543.

[300] Francino, M. P. (Jan 2016). Antibiotics and the Human Gut Microbiome: Dysbioses and Accumulation of Resistances. *Frontiers in Microbiology.* Pubmed, 26793178.

[301] Moloney, R. D.; Desbonnet, L.; Clarke, G.; Dinan, T. G.; & Cryan, J. F. (Feb 2014). The microbiome: stress, health and disease. *Mammalion Genome.* Pubmed, 24281320.

[302] Bi, L.; Triadafilopoulos, G. (Sept 2003). Exercise and gastrointestinal function and disease: an evidence-based review of risks and benefits. *Clinical Gastroenterology Hepatology.* Pubmed, 15017652.

[303] Lee, S. P.; Sung, I.-K.; Kim, J. H.; Lee, S.-Y.; Park, H. S.; & Shim, C. S. (2015). The Effect of Emotional Stress and Depression on the Prevalence of Digestive Diseases. *Journal of Neurogastroenterology and Motility, 21*(2), 273–282. http://doi.org/10.5056/jnm14116

[304] Ansary-Moghaddam, A.; Martiniuk, A.; Lam, T.-H.; Jamrozik, K.; Tamakoshi, A.; Fang, X.; … & Woodward, M. (2009). Smoking and the Risk of Upper Aero Digestive Tract Cancers for Men and Women in the Asia-Pacific Region. *International Journal of Environmental Research and Public Health, 6*(4), 1358–1370. http://doi.org/10.3390/ijerph6041358

[305] Choi, S. Y.; Kahyo, H. (Sept 1991). Effect of cigarette smoking and alcohol consumption in the etiology of cancers of the digestive tract. *International Journal of Cancer.* Pubmed, 1917136.

[306] https://www.stress.org/stress-effects

[307] https://www.stress.org/stress-research

[308] Boone, J. L.; & Anthony, J. P. (2003). Evaluating the impact of stress on systemic disease: the MOST protocol in primary care. *The Journal of the American Osteopathic Association, 103*(5), 239–246.

[309] Lozano, R.; Naghavi, M.; Foreman, K.; Lim, S.; Shibuya, K.; Aboyans, V.; … & AlMazroa, M. A. (2012). Global and regional mortality from 235 causes of death for 20 age groups in 1990 and 2010: a systematic analysis for the Global Burden of Disease Study 2010. *The Lancet, 380*(9859), 2095–2128.

[310] https://www.usatoday.com/story/money/2019/05/28/burnout-official-medical-diagnosis-says-who/1256229001/

[311] Cole, S. W.; Capitanio, J. P.; Chun, K.; Arevalo, J. M.; Ma, J.; & Cacioppo, J. T. (2015). Myeloid differentiation architecture of leukocyte transcriptome dynamics in perceived social isolation. *Proceedings of the National Academy of Sciences, 112*(49), 15142–15147.

312 https://www.economist.com/international/2018/09/01/ loneliness-is-a-serious-public-health-problem

313 https://www.hhs.gov/opioids/about-the-epidemic/opioid-crisis-statistics/ index.html

314 https://www.psychologytoday.com/us/blog/wicked-deeds/201404/ prescription-drugs-are-far-more-deadly-street-drugs

315 https://drugabusestatistics.org/opioid-epidemic/

316 https://www.cdc.gov/drugoverdose/data/statedeaths.html

317 https://www.stress.org/42-worrying-workplace-stress-statistics

318 https://www.stress.org/42-worrying-workplace-stress-statistics

319 Kinnier, R. T.; Hofsess, C.; Pongratz, R.; & Lambert, C. (2009). Attributions and affirmations for overcoming anxiety and depression. *Psychology and Psychotherapy: Theory, Research and Practice, 82*(2), 153–169.

320 Epton, T.; Harris, P. R.; Kane, R.; van Koningsbruggen, G. M.; & Sheeran, P. (2015). The impact of self-affirmation on health-behavior change: A meta-analysis. *Health Psychology, 34*(3), 187.

321 https://www.stress.org/42-worrying-workplace-stress-statistics

322 https://www.wkrn.com/community/health/coronavirus/ cause-of-death-social-isolation-failure-to-thrive-related-to-covid-19-restrictions/

323 https://www.daveramsey.com/blog/bible-verses-about-community

About the Author

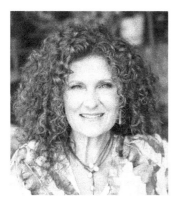

Dani Williamson, MSN, FNP is a Family Nurse Practitioner who is the founder of Integrative Family Medicine, her thriving practice located in Franklin, Tennessee. Dani is living, walking, breathing proof that there is vibrant life after a "lifelong" diagnosis is handed to you.

For decades, Dani suffered from chronic gut issues and autoimmune disease. It wasn't until after graduating from Vanderbilt and working in a naturally minded medical practice that her boss asked her a few life-changing questions: "Dani, what are you eating? Don't you know your diet controls your symptoms?"

Dani did not know this, and she had never heard this during nurse practitioner school. From that moment on, Dani has been on a tireless pursuit to transform her patients' lives through her six steps to healing: eat well, sleep well, move well, poop well, de-stress well, and commune well.

Today, she sees hundreds of patients every month in her clinic and reaches thousands of others through Instagram (Dani Williamson Wellness) as well as her weekly health show on YouTube and Facebook at Dani Williamson Wellness. Her private Facebook community (Inside Out—Healing From Within) has over 10,000 members.

Sign up for her weekly Wild & Well newsletter at
DANIWILLIAMSON.COM/WILD.

Valuable Resources for your Wild & Well Journey!

Stay connected with me and discover recipes and many other resources to aid in your Wild & Well journey.

DANIWILLIAMSON.COM/WILD

I have discounted my online course, "Inflammation is the Devil," for Wild & Well readers only from $199 to just $29. The course is loaded with information and ways to decrease inflammation and accelerate your healing journey.

You can also visit our supplement store online at DaniWlliamson.com, or you can come to the Wild & Well Wellness Emporium in person to check out all of my Wild & Well supplements, hand picked by me. Come by and shop in person six days a week at:

Integrative Family Medicine

330 Mallory Station Road

Franklin, TN 37067

Let's get connected on social media!

Instagram: @daniwilliamsonwellness

YouTube: Dani Williamson Wellness

Facebook: Dani Williamson Wellness

My Instagram is chock full of cooking videos, education, and resources to enhance your life and your wellness journey.

Our daily Facebook live videos discuss important information on supplements and resources designed to help you find healing and joy.

The weekly "Sunday Night Services" on my Dani Williamson Wellness Facebook page (airs @ 6pm CST and on YouTube Monday morning) feature a special guest expert every week. We will bring laugher but more importantly, research and groundbreaking health resources to you each week.

I hope to see you online! And if you are ever in Franklin, stop by the Wild & Well Wellness Emporium supplement store and say hello!

Be Wild & Well!

A free ebook edition
is available with the
purchase of this book.

To claim your free ebook edition:

1. Visit MorganJamesBOGO.com
2. Sign your name CLEARLY in the space
3. Complete the form and submit a photo of the entire copyright page
4. You or your friend can download the ebook to your preferred device

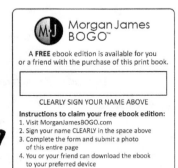

Print & Digital Together Forever.

Snap a photo   Free ebook   Read anywhere

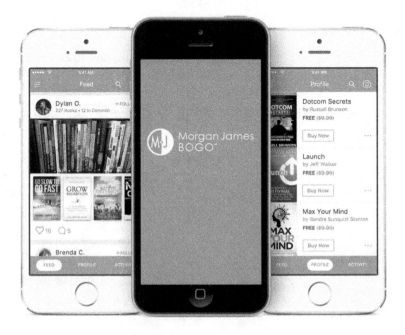